Reflections *on* *Qi*

Reflections on Qi

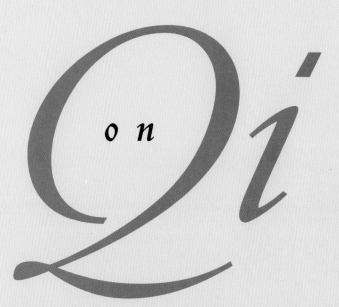

Tuning Your Life to the World's Hidden Energy

Gary Khor

CONTENTS

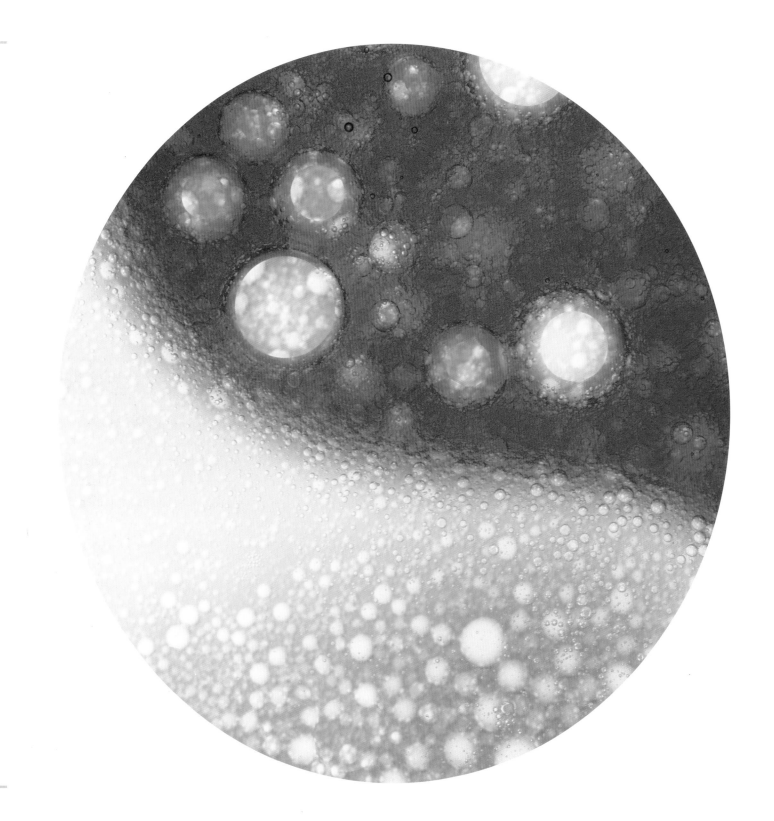

INTRODUCTION

The simple H2O molecule reveals itself to us in many ways: the brilliant beauty of blue-white arctic ice, the mirror finish of a mountain lake, the soft embrace of morning mist or the feather-light touch of a snowflake. We may rejoice in gentle rain or cower during a torrential downpour. Oceans, lakes, rivers, streams, clouds, mist, springs, snow, ice, hail, steam, rainbows and geysers are all simply different ways that we perceive the humble H2O molecule.

This diversity of expression, however, is nothing compared to the diversity exhibited by Qi, for Qi is everything—every type of energy, every type of matter. Everything that we see, hear, touch, feel or detect with our senses or with mechanical instruments is but one of the myriad reflections by which we perceive the underlying Qi. Our very thoughts and emotions, our mind and our consciousness, are but reflections of Qi.

This may sound very mystical, but the search for one basic energy that explains the entire workings of the universe is in fact the 'holy grail' of modern physics. The ancient Chinese, through their concept of Qi, had already arrived at the 'Grand Unification Theory' or 'Theory of Everything', as modern physicists describe their search, millennia ago. However, recognising the existence of a basic universal energy and understanding it are two different things. Sometimes visualising Qi can seem as difficult as trying to visualise the flames of a fire when all you have ever seen of a fire is the flickering light and shadows it has cast upon a wall. While the task is difficult, it is made easier by the observations of the Chinese who over thousands of years sought to gather the clues left in Qi's reflections, and learn to understand something of the seasons, rhythms and currents of this animating power.

Understanding Qi is not simply a pleasant intellectual exercise. The ancient mariners used their knowledge of the currents and rhythms of the oceans to travel more safely upon them and to discover new lands. Today we can use our knowledge of the rhythms and currents of Qi to navigate our way across the energetic ocean that it forms. In doing this our life's voyage will be a little more secure and our lives enriched. Who knows—perhaps we will even reach destinations in life that would otherwise be beyond our reach.

CHAPTER ONE

QI

WHAT IS QI?

It is difficult to translate the word Qi into English. Qi literally means 'breath', but this is less a reference to the mechanical process of respiration than it is to the philosophical concept of breathing life into something. Perhaps the best description of the word Qi is to refer to it as being the 'animating energy' that drives all activity and change within the universe, whether it be associated with living or non-living things.

In one sense Qi is light, sound, heat, emotion, thought, matter and all the other things and processes that exist in the universe. In another sense Qi is none of these things, because each is only an aspect or reflection of Qi. Understanding Qi as the fire behind the universe is a good start. However, we should be careful not to delude ourselves that any description can carry more than a brief glimpse of understanding Qi. Ponder the meaning of the words of Lao Tse, the Chinese philosopher who wrote the *Tao Te Ching* over two-and-a-half millennia ago:

THE WAY THAT CAN BE DESCRIBED IS NOT THE ETERNAL WAY.
THE NAME THAT CAN BE NAMED IS NOT THE ETERNAL NAME.
THE UNNAMEABLE IS THE SOURCE OF THE UNIVERSE.
THE NAMEABLE IS THE SOURCE OF ALL THINGS WITHIN THE UNIVERSE.
CONTEMPLATE THE WAY FOR ITS OWN SAKE AND YOU WILL SEE THE MYSTERY.
CONTEMPLATE THE WAY FOR A PURPOSE AND YOU WILL SEE THE EFFECTS.
MYSTERY AND EFFECTS SPRING FROM THE SAME SOURCE.

The fact that we will never know exactly what Qi is may be a source of frustration for some people. Personally, I am profoundly grateful for the fact that there will always be mystery and wonder within this universe.

If we can never fully understand what Qi is, does this mean we should not study it? Perhaps I can best answer that question by reflecting on the fact that it is unlikely that we will ever fully understand another human being, yet who would sacrifice the enrichment of life that comes from even partial glimpses of the spirit, depth and complexity of those who share our lives?

QI AND MODERN PHYSICS

Modern science currently explains the physical workings of the universe in the terms of four forces: gravity, electromagnetism, the 'strong' nuclear force and the 'weak' nuclear force. It was only relatively recently that 'electricity' and 'magnetism' were understood to be different aspects of the one force of electromagnetism, and most modern physicists believe that future discoveries will eventually result in these four forces being seen simply as aspects of one underlying energy. When modern scientists find their 'Grand Unified Theory' or 'Theory of Everything', modern science and ancient Chinese philosophy will have converged more completely than modern science and ancient Greek philosophy did with atomic theory.

WHERE DOES QI COME FROM?

The Chinese refer to the state that existed before our universe was born as 'Wu Qi' which can be roughly translated as the 'pregnant void'. This poetic description captures the belief that Wu Qi contained within it the potential for all things, for every type of universe that could exist—whatever physical laws that universe was built on. Rather than the Big Bang theory of the western world, the Chinese believe that the process starts with what we might call 'The Great Separation', the separating forces of yin and yang.

As a modern analogy look at what happens when you throw a switch to create an electric circuit. There is an immediate creation of a negative and a positive flow of energy. Think of the positive current that fires up the universe as the yang force, and the negative current as the yin force. The interplay of positive and negative then create all of the interactions and processes that we see around us in the universe. Through the differentiation of yin and yang, Qi (the energy that was always there) can be seen in action as the force that drives yin and yang to transform and balance each other.

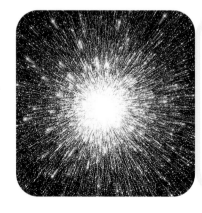

The Big Bang theory maintains that the expansion and consequent cooling of the universe allowed matter to coalesce out of this energy, interact in subatomic and chemical reactions and become more and more complex, producing the universe we see around us today. But whereas the Big Bang theory predicts the eventual collapse or running down of the universe, Qi theory is much more optimistic—there seems no reason why the great dance of yin and yang should ever stop. Even if it does, in Chinese terms the death of our universe would simply be a return to Wu Qi and a re-creation of the pregnant void from which all things become possible.

IS QI ALL THERE IS?

The concept of Qi is not sufficient of itself. Qi behaves in certain ways and this behaviour must be governed by the equivalent of physical laws, which the Chinese refer to as 'Li', or 'principle'. Qi behaves in accordance with Li, which creates the pattern of Qi. The interaction of Li and Qi creates the 'Tao', or the way. Li is a very important concept within Traditional Chinese thinking, but it should not be confused with the word 'Li' in Confucian terminology, which refers to etiquette or ritual.

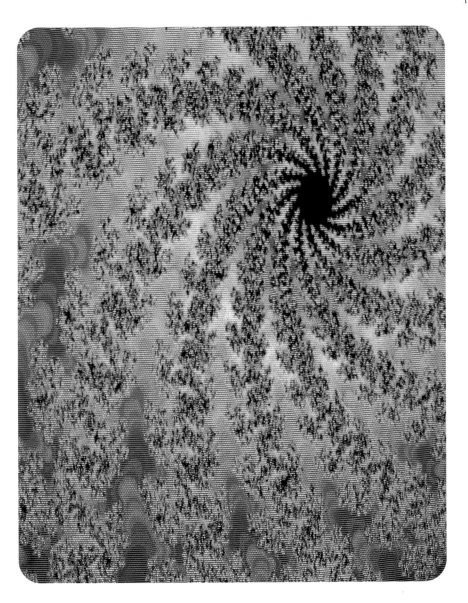

Modern chaos theory has shown that within apparent chaos there is infinite order. Li may be thought of as the pattern that underlies the universe as we perceive it. This pattern is not static but evolves through time—this is the role of Qi.

Think of a kaleidoscope. A beautiful pattern is created by reflecting mirrors which in effect 'order' the pattern. If you then shake the kaleidoscope, the pattern changes. This can be likened to the animating force of Qi. While every pattern looks different, each will have the same number of segments as every other pattern. In that sense Li determines the nature of the pattern.

This seems to be what we are discovering about the nature of chaos itself. We can go deeper and deeper into the pattern but its basic nature always remains the same. In one sense, when we discover some deep mathematical relationship or equation that seems to describe the universe, what we are doing is discovering part of the pattern that is Li.

WORKING WITH QI

Working with a universal force like Qi can seem a bit daunting. Relax. Every time you do something as simple as choosing a site for a plant in your garden you are working with the light energy generated by the vast thermonuclear reactions of the sun. You will be able to do a lot to ensure the proper positioning and health of that plant without understanding anything about thermonuclear reactions, photons, wavelengths of light and so on. This analogy demonstrates that working with powerful, complex systems can be quite simple.

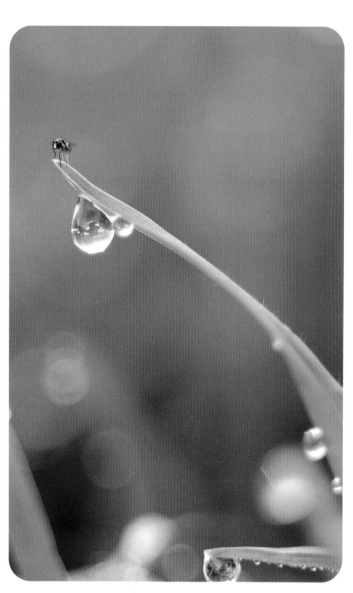

What we might call the 'underlying Qi' and the 'expression of Qi' that we perceive in our everyday reality are two sides of the same coin. You cannot have a change in one without a change in the other. Just as your thoughts, emotions, health and relationships are products of the 'underlying Qi', changes in those same things can change the nature of the 'underlying Qi'.

Does this imply that any change you make to the 'expressions of Qi' around you must have been due to changes that were going on in the underlying Qi in the first place? Is there no point in trying to make changes to Qi since these changes will either happen or not happen regardless of our involvement? This is a restatement of those problems of predestiny and free will that philosophers have wrestled with since the beginning of recorded history. (On a religious level the problem can be restated as, 'If our creator already knows the future, then in what sense can we have free will?') Personally I view these problems simply as deficiencies in the way that our minds grasp the world.

The traditional Chinese were pragmatic people. They saw that when they effected certain changes in their lifestyle the expression of the underlying nature of Qi itself changed, so they created a number of arts to work with Qi, including:

- MEDICAL QIGONG—WITH A FOCUS ON REBALANCING THE INTERNAL QI FOR HEALING PURPOSES.

- HEALTH QIGONG—WITH A FOCUS ON DEVELOPING HEALTH AND VITALITY AND INCREASING LONGEVITY.

- MARTIAL ARTS QIGONG—WITH A FOCUS ON USING QI TO INCREASE POWER AND AWARENESS.

- SPIRITUAL QIGONG—WITH A FOCUS ON REFINING AND DEVELOPING QI AS A MEANS OF SPIRITUAL PROGRESSION AND ALIGNMENT.

- SEXUAL QIGONG—WITH A FOCUS ON THE USE OF SEXUAL PRACTICES TO DEVELOP AND ENHANCE QI.

- PERFORMANCE QIGONG—WITH A FOCUS ON ENHANCING FITNESS AND PERFORMANCE IN SPORTS.

- ENVIRONMENTAL QIGONG (FENG SHUI)—WITH A FOCUS ON USING THE QI CONTAINED WITHIN THE ENVIRONMENT ITSELF, ALONG WITH TECHNIQUES FOR MODIFYING IT, TO ENSURE THAT A PERSON'S QI IS SUPPORTED BY THE QI OF THEIR ENVIRONMENT.

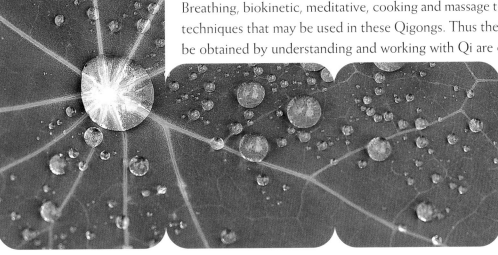

Breathing, biokinetic, meditative, cooking and massage techniques are just some of the techniques that may be used in these Qigongs. Thus the the range of benefits that can be obtained by understanding and working with Qi are enormous.

THE WAVES OF QI

Our world is full of waves. We see them on the ocean, on windblown grass and in the leaves of trees. (The Chinese even have different names for the types of wave motion in the leaves of trees, such as 'pine waves' and 'willow waves'.) We speak casually of 'sound waves' and 'radio waves'. Scientists understand the whole electromagnetic spectrum simply as waves whose different frequencies generate the colours that we see around us and a range of other energies, such as X rays and microwaves. Earthquakes occur when waves pass through the very ground itself. All materials resonate (pass waves through themselves) to some degree, which is why you hear an approaching train better when you place your ears against the metal rails. Scientists are now even looking for 'gravity waves'.

The Chinese were fascinated by the cycles that they found almost everywhere in nature. When such cycles are plotted as graphs their inherent wave nature is revealed. The frequency with which Qi manifests itself in the form of waves suggests that this reflects some deep aspect of the underlying nature of Qi. Indeed, the Chinese deeply study and examine these repetitious wave patterns on the basis that they can be used to predict the future. The *I Ching* (Chinese book of divination) is based on the 64 phases through which Qi passes, each stage having a specific energy configuration and thus specific occurrences and trends associated

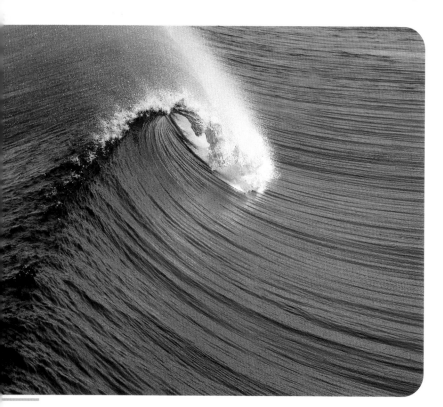

with it. The Chinese view of the future is not that it is fixed and that 'you are going to meet a tall dark stranger on so and so day'; it is more like forecasting the weather and arranging your activities in accordance with what suits the predicted weather patterns.

Most cultures observe energetic patterns to some degree. Even something as basic as predicting the wave pattern of the seasons allows us to plan our holidays and predict the type of clothes we will need at certain times. The Chinese have simply made such a reading an art form.

In the modern economy no-one finds it strange that 'Chartists' plot the rhythms in the movement of stock market values in order to predict the appropriate times at which to buy and sell. Indeed, business people rarely prosper if they do not understand the 'business cycle', another rhythm or wave-like pattern that pulses throughout our world.

THE MANY NAMES OF QI

You may see Qi written in many different ways—Qi, Chi, Ki, Chee, Ke and Khe—and you may see the word attached to many different modifiers such as: Yin Qi, Yang Qi, Sha Qi, Si Qi, Sheng Qi, Heart Qi, Liver Qi, Kidney Qi, Yuan Qi, Fire Qi, Water Qi, Wood Qi, etc etc. This can sometimes be a little confusing, particularly when you read again and again that there is only one Qi. The different spellings of Qi have arisen simply because it is very difficult to get a phonetic rendition of the Chinese pronunciation of the word Qi in western languages. None of the different spellings of the word Qi has any significance at all. The closest phonetic rendition might actually be 'Khee'.

Modifiers are added to the word Qi because 'underlying Qi' may reflect itself through many different aspects of the physical world, and the speaker or writer needs to indicate which particular aspect or perspective he or she has on Qi at that time. This may include the quantity, location, source, rate of movement, phase or function of Qi at any point in time. When you think about it, this is no more mysterious than us having different names for H2O molecules depending on how many of them we have in one place—a drop, puddle, pond, pool, lake, sea or ocean. Or what 'state' those molecules are in—snow, ice, rain, cloud, steam, mist, frost, icicles, sleet or hail.

Another thing that may cause confusion is that Ren Qi, the name given to the Qi within human beings, is often abbreviated to Qi because the context makes it clear (to the Chinese) what aspect of Qi is being referred to. Ren Qi must be understood as that Qi which signifies human life. It is itself a division of Hwo Qi, the Qi that makes living things living. When something is dead it still has its own kind of Qi, but this is known as Syy Qi or Goe Qi (ghost Qi).

Human Qi (Ren Qi) is one of the three major divisions of Qi, along with Heaven Qi (Tien Qi) and Earth Qi (Ti Qi).

THE STATES OF QI

Most of us are familiar with the concept that matter can exist in different states such as solid, liquid or gas. (Other states, such as plasma and the degenerate matter that exist in places such as neutron stars and white dwarfs, may not be quite as familiar.) Most of us are not, however, used to thinking of energy as existing in different states. We tend to think of all energy as one amorphous state of being.

However, if we accept the fact that matter can assume quite different properties simply because of the degree of association between different atoms or subatomic particles, why should we be surprised if different states of energy should turn out to have quite different properties? Science speaks of energy states such as energy currents (the flows within an electric wire or down the ionised channel of a lightning bolt, for example) and energy fields (such as gravity fields and magnetic fields). We can also learn that electricity currents create electromagnetic fields and that moving electro-magnetic fields generate currents. This type of knowledge has considerable relevance to the understanding of Qi, for newcomers to the study of traditional Chinese medicine are often confused by the fact that Qi sometimes behaves like an energy field (as in Wei Qi, the body's defensive energy, or Shen Qi, the body's spirit or vitality) and sometimes behaves like a current of energy (as in the body's meridians or the use of Jing Qi in martial arts). If energy works as an interaction of currents and fields in the universe at large, we should be surprised if it does not work that way in the human body too.

Mystics have long spoken of different vibrational levels and 'planes of existence'. Perhaps in part what they were talking about was different 'states' of energy. Certainly the traditional Chinese have long held that Qi can be transmuted into different states. This is very similar in fact to the Hindu 'chakra' concept, where body energy centres of various vibrational frequencies are associated with various 'spiritual' states. The Chinese tend to relate these centres to different emotions and health conditions, though spiritual quality does come into it at deeper levels.

What we are talking about here is no more wondrous than the fact that changing the frequency of visible light in turn changes its colour and may even change its nature into such things as microwaves, radio waves, X-rays and other parts of the electromagnetic spectrum. We might also speculate whether thought, emotion and spirit should be regarded simply as different states of energy which are as inevitable as gravity and as integral to the nature of the universe. We are likely to be just as offended by the suggestion that the building blocks of our emotions, thought and spirit are to be found in every rock and grain of sand as we once were by the concept that the plants and animals around us all shared a common origin. Then again, many cultures, including Australia's Aboriginal culture—the oldest culture on Earth—have long held the view that their land embodies these very attributes.

THE HISTORY OF QI

How long ago did the Chinese formulate the concept of Qi? There is much controversy about the subject. The Chinese were content to accept that the concepts could be traced back to the time of the three sovereigns, commencing around 2850BCE. Western scholars initially felt that this might have been overly imaginative, and regarded the three sovereigns more as mythical figures than real. However, it now appears that the Chinese may have been too conservative in their estimates of the antiquity of their beliefs. Each new archaeological discovery seems to push back the dates and show evidence that the Qi theory has an amazing antiquity. As we shall learn in chapter two, the yin-yang concept was formulated to explain the workings of Qi. One of the ways that the yin-yang concept is depicted is through the symbol of a conflict between a dragon and a tiger (see page 36). A Neolithic burial site dated at 5000BCE contains these symbols.

Certainly stone probes called Bian Shyr were used to adjust Qi circulation. These have been found in Shang dynasty (1766–1154BCE) archaeological digs. Such Qi adjustment techniques would indicate considerable development of the theory at that date. The *I Ching* (Chinese book of divination), one of the most sophisticated applications of Qi theory, is ascribed to the year 1122BCE.

CHAPTER TWO

THE TAO OF

QI

The Tao of Qi could be partially rendered in English as the 'Way of Energy', the 'Road' that energy takes. This road is made visible in the universe that surrounds us, for that world is no more and no less than a physical expression of the Tao of Qi.

Since our universe was created it has become more intricate and richer in its diversity, yet the physical laws that support this diversity are the same as they were at the moment of its creation, when only the one uniform energy state existed (apart from the breathtakingly small irregularities postulated by modern astrophysicists). Is this a Tao of Qi that things grow ever more diverse and complex? Do we see the same thing happen with life on Earth, with human language, with society, with the computer programs that form our software? Do those who aspire to the monolithic, the universal political state, the empire that will last 10 000 years, recognise that the universe does not work that way?

Everything is destined to die, be it a person, a business, a nation, a species or the very planet we live on. So is the Tao of Qi a Tao of futility? Or should we ask, 'What if the initial state of the universe had lasted forever? What if the day never died because the Earth faced the sun eternally? What if the seasons never changed? What if the first life form never evolved?' Would this have resulted in a universe more to our liking? Hardly, for we would never have existed to make such an evaluation. The truth is that nothing dies and that one pattern of energy transforms into another. The Tao of Qi is the Tao of Transformation.

In the world around us there are seasons and cycles, currents in the air and oceans and currents in the tide of human life. The Tao of Qi is to flow and ebb. We can ride those currents or fight those currents, but if we are to do either successfully, we must know and understand those currents. We must know the Tao of Qi.

QI AND THE HARMONY OF YIN AND YANG

We learned in the previous chapter that Qi operates in accordance with certain laws or principles called Li, and that there is a pattern, a rhythm, a current to Qi. Without knowledge of how Qi flows and how these flows manifest themselves in the universe, Qi is simply an intellectual abstraction. Understand those flows and you are a sailor who understands the currents of wind and water, where your destination lies, where the currents hold opportunities and where they hold threats. This is an infinitely better proposition than being swept this way and that by unknown and unpredictable forces.

What we need is the equivalent of a compass—an instrument that will unerringly point to the direction in which the Qi is flowing, regardless of the actual direction that we want to go in. The yin-yang concept provides us with such an intellectual instrument.

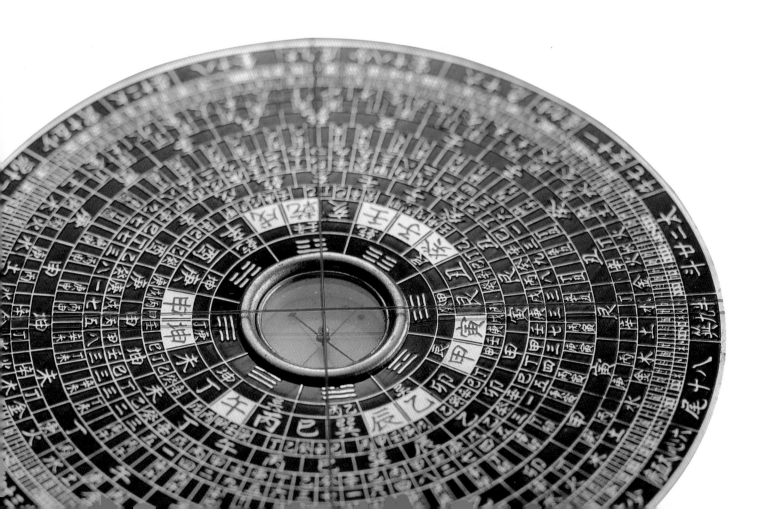

WHAT IS QIGONG?

Gong or kung literally means 'work' so Qigong is work with Qi. Since one of the meanings of Qi is 'breath', one more limited use of the term is 'breath work', as used in breathing for meditation and health purposes. In China the term is used much more widely, to encompass any activity that is used to enhance the flow of Qi within the human body either to improve health or to achieve some exterior objective (such as painting a picture, creating calligraphy, etc).

The two broad divisions of Qigong are known as Nei Dan Qigong (Internal Qigong) and Wei Dan Qigong (External Qigong). The meanings of these terms may vary depending on the level of activity being referred to. When the term Wei Dan Qigong is used with regard to health exercise systems or martial arts it refers to the systems that work on developing the raw muscular power of the body. These in turn are often termed 'Shaolin' in reference to the temple where the development of forms of this nature reached their peak. Nei Dan Qigong works on the development of the internal power of the body through the removal of all stress and tension and the development of internal health. Tai Chi Chuan, Hsing I and Ba Kua are the forms people are most familiar with.

Nei Dan Qigong includes all of the above forms plus any system that uses the internal resources of the body. Wei Dan Qigongs are those with a focus that lies outside the body, such as Qi nutrition, Feng Shui and health arts applied by another person (acumassage, moxabustion and so forth).

To understand more about the nature of Qigong let us look at the difference between doing a physical exercise and practising a physical Qigong form.

Performing a physical exercise involves nothing more than burning calories by using the muscles. I often see people on exercise bikes peddling furiously while reading a book, with little interest or involvement in the movement they are making. Undoubtably they are getting exercise, but for such an exercise to become a Qigong the body's physical, emotional, intellectual and energetic aspects would need to be involved. Thus, in a Qigong:

- ALL MUSCULAR 'STRESS' WITHIN THE BODY IS RELEASED. ONE MUST DISTINGUISH BETWEEN THE MUSCLE 'TENSION' THAT IS UNNECESSARY FOR THE PERFORMANCE OF THE EXERCISE AND THE MUSCULAR ACTIVITY NECESSARY TO CARRY OUT THE EXERCISE. THIS TECHNIQUE IS CALLED 'SUNG' AND INVOLVES 'SINKING THE QI' (SEE PAGE 59).

- • - The posture should support the flow of Qi throughout the body. This involves the 'suspended headtop' technique for proper alignment of the spine as well as the 'Mian' (silk-like) movement where the joints are kept open (see page 59).

- • - The breath should be relaxed and diaphragmatic.

- • - The intellectual mind should be focused on maintaining a particular rhythm or speed.

- • - The emotional mind should be calm and relaxed, enjoying the sensory input that performance of the movement brings.

APPROACHING THE YIN-YANG CONCEPT

The terms 'yin' and 'yang' are so fundamental to the understanding of Qi and so much a foundation of traditional Chinese thinking that it is essential that the terms be understood and used correctly. This is much easier for those brought up within traditional Chinese culture, where one absorbs the meanings and subtleties of these concepts from a thousand different associations and applications, simply through the ordinary process of living. To distill all this into a few paragraphs of writing risks oversimplifying and missing the full meaning of the terms. To appreciate the problem I challenge you to perform a little thought experiment: imagine that you have a visitor from another world and they ask you to explain to them what the word 'love' means. Despite the fact that you have heard and used this word thousands of times I suspect that you may find it a little difficult to explain the term. Sometimes, it seems, a term can only be understood, not explained.

Being brought up in a traditional Chinese cultural framework makes it easier to understanding the term 'yin-yang'. For those of us who do not have this opportunity, another way is to explore traditional Chinese techniques and arts, letting each of them provide a number of glimpses or insights into the yin-yang concept that will gradually build up into a full understanding. In this part of the book I have therefore sought to provide you with a basic conceptual framework. While this may seem somewhat abstract and theoretical, it is my hope that as you move through this book and apply the concepts to your body, mind, health, environment, diet and daily activities, you will begin to understand what a brilliantly universal, useful tool the yin-yang concept is.

THE YIN-YANG SYMBOL

The yin-yang symbol represents two mutually dependent aspects of energy whose interaction is the animating power of the universe. The yin aspect of energy or Qi is represented by a darker colour (usually black but sometimes blue) that expands in size as it moves down. The yang aspect of energy is represented by a lighter colour (usually white but sometimes red) that expands in size as it moves up. Both aspects take up half of the area of a circle making them equal in size and shape. Within each of the yin-yang aspects is a small dot with a colour representing the opposite aspect. This is to symbolise the fact that even as each aspect reaches the height of its power it carries within it the seed of the other aspect.

As we continue our exploration of the yin-yang concept you will see just how sophisticated this symbolic representation of the concept is. Niels Bohr, the founder of modern atomic theory, included the symbol in his family crest because he could think of no other symbol that better explained how the universe worked. You will often see the symbol used as a good luck charm in the Chinese art of Feng Shui. This is because it represents balance and harmony within life, and such balance and harmony is believed to promote happiness and success.

THE ORIGINAL MEANINGS OF YIN AND YANG

The terms yin and yang were first used to describe the two sides of a mountain. Yang was the description given to the sunny side, while yin was the description given to the shady side of that mountain. Of course no mountain has a permanent yin or yang side, for as the sun rises and falls the shady side becomes the sunny side and vice versa.

To make this description even more useful, instead of thinking of yin and yang as terms describing the relative amounts of light present on the two sides of the mountain, let us think of this as a shorthand way of describing the relative amounts of energy present on the two sides of the mountain.

For now, we will treat the yang side of our mountain as being the more energetic side and the yin as the less energetic side. So:

- WITH REGARD TO TEMPERATURE, THE HOTTER SIDE OF THE MOUNTAIN WILL BE THE YANG SIDE AND THE COLDER SIDE THE YIN.

- WITH REGARD TO SOUND, THE LOUDER SIDE OF THE MOUNTAIN WILL BE THE YANG SIDE AND THE QUIETER SIDE THE YIN.

- WITH REGARD TO MOISTURE, THE DRYER SIDE OF THE MOUNTAIN WILL BE THE YANG SIDE AND THE WETTER SIDE THE YIN.

- WITH REGARD TO ACTIVITY AND MOVEMENT, THE SIDE WITH MORE ACTIVITY AND MOVEMENT WILL BE THE YANG SIDE AND THE SIDE WITH LESS ACTIVITY AND MOVEMENT THE YIN.

Thus any energetic characteristic of matter can be used to tell us whether, in terms of that characteristic, the object is yin or yang in respect to another object.

This, however, is only the more obvious part of the story. To the Chinese, all things are reflections of Qi, and everything has its yin-yang polarity, including matter. In fact one may consider matter as simply semi-permanent patterns of energy (or Qi). To understand yin-yang concepts in terms of matter let us compare two mountains rather than two sides of one mountain:

- WITH REGARD TO HEIGHT, THE HIGHEST MOUNTAIN WILL BE THE YANG MOUNTAIN AND THE LOWEST MOUNTAIN THE YIN MOUNTAIN.

- WITH REGARD TO SHAPE, THE SHARPEST, MOST ANGULAR MOUNTAIN WILL BE THE YANG MOUNTAIN AND THE LEAST SHARP, LEAST ANGULAR MOUNTAIN THE YIN MOUNTAIN.

- WITH REGARD TO HARDNESS OR ROUGHNESS, THE HARDEST, ROUGHEST MOUNTAIN WILL BE THE YANG MOUNTAIN AND THE SOFTEST, SMOOTHEST MOUNTAIN THE YIN MOUNTAIN.

Thus any physical characteristic of matter can be used to tell us whether, in terms of that characteristic, the object is yin or yang in respect to another object.

MONO-'QI'-ISM

When we apply yin-yang concepts to different physical and energetic aspects we must be very careful not to fall into the trap of thinking that there is a Qi of light or a Qi of shape. There is only one underlying Qi, of which we catch different glimpses in the form of light and shape. Retaining this understanding is essential when we come to putting the yin-yang concept to practical effect in our everyday life.

A simple thought experiment shows us that there is no difference between Qi that has a yang effect and Qi that has a yin effect.

Imagine you have three beakers of water—one contains a goldfish swimming peacefully, one is filled with ice, and the third is boiling vigorously.

When the beaker of ice water is compared with the beaker that contains the goldfish, the ice water beaker is yin compared with the warmer water of the goldfish beaker, which in comparison is yang. When the beaker of boiling water is compared with the beaker with the goldfish swimming in it, then the boiling water beaker is yang compared to the goldfish beaker, which in comparison is yin.

The Qi that underlies the goldfish beaker does not change depending on whether it is being compared with hotter or colder water; the same Qi can have a yin or yang effect depending on the relative energy state of the item it is being compared to. There is no Yin Qi or Yang Qi. There is only Qi.

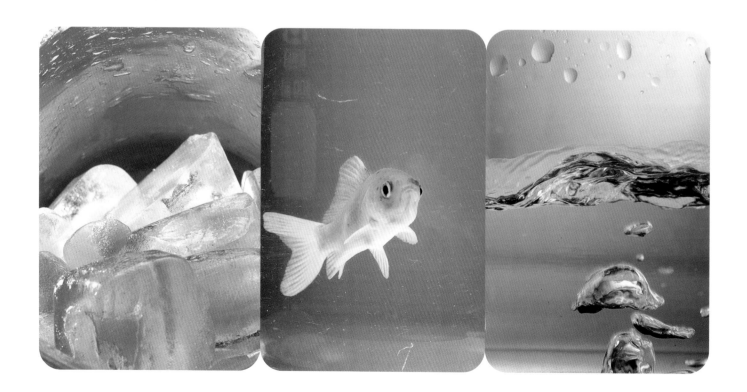

THE VALLEY PRINCIPLE

If you think you are starting to get the hang of this, consider that when comparing two mountains:

- •- WITH REGARD TO MASS, THE MOST MASSIVE MOUNTAIN WILL IN FACT BE THE YIN MOUNTAIN AND THE LEAST MASSIVE MOUNTAIN THE YANG MOUNTAIN.

At first this may seem counter-intuitive but it is an important part of understanding the yin-yang concept. Yin is seen as the source of energy, that which gathers and collects together to accumulate energy, whereas yang is seen as the expenditure of energy, that which is dispersive and expansive. In terms of the above example, a mountain that is smaller than another mountain is smaller for one of two reasons: it never 'collected' together as much material when it was first formed or more of its material has dispersed due to erosion.

In either event, the underlying Qi of the most massive mountain represents energy that is more yin in nature than the underlying Qi that represents the frozen energy of the less massive mountain. If this sounds like a purely mystical statement consider the situation from a scientific perspective.

Science knows that mountains are created by geological forces that raise certain parts of the Earth's crust. Generally this is through movements of continental plates or through volcanic action. The amount of energy that must be used to raise a mountain depends largely on the mass of the material within it. The mountain with more mass has more potential energy (kinetic energy of position) bound up within it. If the mountain is smaller because of subsequent erosion, then in effect the potential energy of position has been transformed into other energies, as the mountain's material has been removed by the agents of wind, water and gravity. In this way the original potential energy has been removed and the mountain now has less potential energy (less yin) in comparison with the more massive mountain. Saying that something is less yin than something else is another way of saying that it is more yang.

If it appears that I am labouring this point it is to prevent a common misconception that can arise concerning the nature of yin and yang, and thus the nature of Qi. That misconception is that when something is yin in comparison to something else it has less Qi, when in fact something that is yin expends less Qi (and therefore gathers more Qi).

This is why the traditional Chinese extol the yin or 'valley' principle. Yin is the source of yang. If a yin process does not exist and accumulate the Qi that a yang process is expending, the result is exhaustion and depletion. To go back to our example, unless the mountain-building activity continues (through the yin process), our glorious mountain will eventually be eroded (by the yang process) until it becomes flat, featureless bedrock. As a practical illustration of the effects of this principle the ancient Chinese noted that in the high alpine ranges the valleys were filled with lush undergrowth and good farming land, making them a desirable place to live. The higher up the mountain they went though, the more exposed they were to storms and wind, the more sparse the vegetation and the less useful the land was for farming.

If you wanted exhilaration and stimulation then you went mountain climbing. If you wanted to live a pleasant, comfortable life you lived in those areas that represented the accumulation of energy, not the expenditure of energy. In general, if you were seeking harmony you looked for the energetic valleys, not the energetic mountains.

It is interesting to reflect on how the yin-yang nature of our culture impacts on our perception of mountains. We have a particularly yang culture at the moment. You can't get a much more yang symbol than a sharp, jagged mountain outline, and our culture today loves the sight of these dramatic-looking mountains. Yet during the Victorian age mountains were generally depicted in art as dark, looming, sinister, threatening landscapes. I recall reading a travelogue written in this period by a traveller passing through Switzerland who would pull down the blinds on his coach when confronted with the sight of mountains because the sight of them made him physically ill. The interesting thing is that from his writing he obviously saw this as a no more unusual response than becoming seasick.

Another thing that might be bothering you is why the Taoists—the greatest followers of the valley principle—built their monasteries and temples on mountains. Well, as we shall see in chapter five, it all depends on the specific effect you want the energy of your environment to have on the energy of your life.

YIN-YANG TRANSFORMATION POWERS THE UNIVERSE

On a cosmic scale the universe only began to 'run' when Qi split into its negative and positive aspects, its yin and yang polarities. In Chinese terms the 'great split' provided the energy for the Big Bang. One is reminded of the flood of energy that is released when we split the atom. Scientists now suspect that there is much more energy in pure vacuum than there ever is in matter, and that if we could somehow split nothing we might end up with more energy than we could handle!

anti-matter

Less cosmic scales are easier to grasp so let's return for the moment to the analogy we drew in chapter one between Qi and electricity (see page 16). An electric circuit must contain both a positive and a negative flow of electricity or there is no current and no work done in terms of powering a light bulb, refrigerator, computer or television. The negative yin energy flow and the positive yang energy flow can be seen as the electric circuits through which Qi flows to power every activity and transformation that takes place within the universe.

It is important to recognise that the electrons do not change in themselves as they pass from the positive to the negative part of the circuit; they only change what they are doing. (In the positive wire case they move outwards to the source of the work—the electric light filament for example—and in the negative wire they move back to the source of the current.) If you could somehow extract one electron from the positive wire and one electron from the negative wire and compare them you would find no difference. Likewise, if you compared an electron from a direct current circuit and an alternating current circuit you would find no distinction. So whether Qi is having a yin or a yang effect it is the same Qi—it is simply travelling in a different direction.

Perhaps the most important thing to understand is that the moving out and the moving back direction of electrons are equally important to the doing of the work by the electric current. Think of Newton's third law, 'For every action there is an equal and opposite reaction.' You cannot have one without the other. You may think that a rocket flies from the 'action' of throwing out a jet of expansive propellant, but it is in fact the 'reaction' to this that lifts the rocket.

Our electric circuit analogy is good in another sense too because we know that the wires must be able to carry the same amount of electricity, for the positive and negative flows must balance!

So this analogy is a reminder of three important things:

- •- YIN AND YANG ARE SIMPLY TWO ASPECTS OF THE SAME QI.

- •- BOTH YIN AND YANG MUST BE PRESENT FOR WORK TO BE DONE.

- •- OVER TIME YIN AND YANG WILL MOVE TOWARDS BALANCE.

PUTTING THE YIN-YANG CONCEPT TO WORK

Now all this discussion is intellectually interesting but why is it practically important? The reason the Chinese wanted to classify things as yin and yang in relation to each other was because it allowed them to predict the energetic effect one would have on the other—they could then manipulate their environment with confidence to achieve the energetic effects they wanted.

In modern science a similar but more limited concept is contained within the laws of thermodynamics, which state that when you have two energy states of different levels the energy states tend to equalise (ie pour hot water into cold water and you end up with warm water). Since, as the laws of thermodynamics also state, 'energy can neither be created nor destroyed', if a system is converting energy to work then eventually that system must run down. These depressing laws, while of vital importance in engineering and in understanding how processes in the universe work, predict the running down or heat-death of the entire universe.

I mention this because while the laws of thermodynamics can be contained within the yin-yang concept, the yin-yang concept cannot be contained within the laws of thermo-dynamics. In essence the laws of thermodynamics recognise only the yang processes of the universe, that is, those that (on a universal time scale) dissipate energy. There is no recognition of a universal yin principle. This is one reason why modern science cannot explain the origins of the universe: it contains no creative yin element within its theory. Yin conditions are always seen as temporary aberrations of a yang process, rather than a fundamental process in their own right.

We can extend the concept that mixing hot and cold results in warm to the more general yin-yang characteristics:

- • - MIXING A DRY SUBSTANCE WITH A WET SUBSTANCE RESULTS IN A MOIST SUBSTANCE.

- • - MIXING AN ANGULAR SHAPE WITH A CURVED SHAPE SOFTENS THE ANGULAR SHAPE AND SHARPENS THE CURVED SHAPE.

- • - MIXING A VISCOUS LIQUID WITH A NON-VISCOUS LIQUID RESULTS IN A SEMI-VISCOUS LIQUID.

- • - MIXING A DARK COLOUR WITH A LIGHT COLOUR LIGHTENS THE DARK COLOUR AND DARKENS THE LIGHT COLOUR.

And so on.

What we are seeing here are glimpses of an underlying universal principle: yin and yang transform each other. If our health, our emotions, our life, our culture or our environment get out of balance, we can use the yin-yang concept to determine the nature of that imbalance and we can also use the concept to identify the means by which that imbalance can be corrected.

Let us suppose, for instance, that we have a conflict situation between two human beings. Such conflict would be an indication of an underlying energy with a yang imbalance. Logic as well as yin-yang theory would tell us that if we are going to use a third party to help calm the situation, that third party's mental state should be calmer than that of the two antagonists. Yin-yang theory, however, tells us much more. It would predict that the situation is much more likely to be brought into balance if:

- • - THE ENVIRONMENT IS MADE MORE YIN. THAT IS, IF THE COLOURS ARE GENERALLY SOFT AND SUBDUED, IF THE SOUNDS ARE MELLOW, IF THE LIGHT LEVEL IS LOWER, IF THE FURNISHINGS ARE SOFT, CURVED AND COMFORTABLE.

- • - ACTIVITIES OF THE ANTAGONISTS ARE MADE MORE YIN. THERE IS MUCH MORE LIKELIHOOD THAT THE CONFLICT WILL BE RESOLVED IF THE PARTIES ARE SITTING RATHER THAN STANDING, IF THEY PARK THE CAR THEY ARE TRAVELLING IN RATHER THAN CONTINUING TO DRIVE, IF THEY SIT DOWN TO A MEAL RATHER THAN SPRING-CLEAN THE HOUSE. LOWERING ENERGY LEVELS THROUGH PHYSICAL ACTIVITY MAY ALSO HELP, BUT NOT IF THE CONFLICT RESOLUTION PROCESS IS ATTEMPTED DURING THE PHYSICAL ACTIVITY.

SHA QI, SI QI AND SHENG QI

While we know from psychological studies and conflict resolution experience that many of the above techniques work, isn't it fascinating that they are all predicted by yin-yang theory? When you read about using yin-yang concepts to help resolve conflict you may have thought, 'Is this man seriously trying to tell me that the best way to resolve conflict is to plunge the room into pitch darkness and absolute silence and have the antagonists lie unmoving on a water bed?' Unfortunately, it is a very common western approach to draw such conclusions. In the art of Feng Shui the Chinese evolved the terms Sha Qi, Si Qi and Sheng Qi, which can be usefully applied throughout any yin-yang discussion to avoid falling into extremism.

The meanings of the terms are often explained through the following analogy. Visualise a peaceful garden stream. The fresh water splashes and gurgles at some points and forms placid pools at others. Plants grow bountifully along the banks and fish and other aquatic life thrive in the water. If we understand that the water represents Qi, then we see that there is just the right amount of Qi to support the perfect stream. We refer to this situation as the state of Sheng Qi.

Let us suppose that a drought comes along. The flow of water slows and stops, algae takes over the surface, mosquitoes thrive, the healthy plants and animals die and rot and a putrid stench fills the air. This is the state of Si Qi, where the quantity and flow of Qi is too small.

On the other hand, suppose that instead of drought it rains day after day. The stream becomes a torrent, the aquatic life and plants are washed away, and the banks begin to collapse and wash away. Eventually the stream overspills its banks, ravages the garden and even threatens the foundations of the house. This is the state of Sha Qi, where the flow of energy is too strong and too fast.

In all instances the stream was just water; it was the quantity of that water and the speed with which it moved that made a vital difference to the environment that we sought. In the same way there is a range of Qi that is appropriate for any activity. If we move out of that range in either direction the activity is not supported.

In our example of conflict resolution, dimming the lights was appropriate but complete elimination of light, which would create a Si Qi situation, was not. Otherwise the energy to support the conflict would not be present, but neither would the energy to support the process of conflict resolution. Similarly, while depression can often be overcome by raising the energy level of activities and the environment, getting a depressed person to run a marathon then sit with bright interrogation lights shining in their eyes is not recommended. We must always make our yin-yang adjustments within the range that falls within Sheng Qi. Identifying the Sheng Qi range is the real art of the Qigong master.

COMMON MISCONCEPTIONS ABOUT THE YIN-YANG CONCEPT

You may have heard that females are yin in comparison with males. Understandably, feminists are often annoyed when they hear that they are associated with aspects of the body rather than aspects of the mind, and that yin is submissive and yang is assertive. But the yin-yang concept certainly does not foist on the female population the concept that the true female is a submissive, less intelligent person who is more tied up in the senses than the intellect.

'Left' is considered yin when compared with 'right', 'lower' is considered yin when compared with 'upper', and 'back' is considered yin when compared with 'front', but this does not mean that the true female comes with no upper, right or back half. Each yin-yang couplet is independent. Just because one attribute is yin doesn't mean that all attributes will be yin, just as something that is bright is not necessarily 'hot' (as those who have suffered snow-blindness know). The 'female principle' that we often hear about in yin-yang theory is a simple reference to the procreative act involving the process of receiving and generating—it is not a suggestion that a human female must consist of entirely yin characteristics, nor that a human male must be overactive, aggressive and unfeeling.

When applied to human beings, the yin-yang concept is always about creating harmony and balance. Yin-yang couplets contain no value judgements and there is no 'dark side of the force'.

QI AND THE HARMONY OF THE FIVE ELEMENTS

The yin-yang concept gives us a most powerful tool with which to study and use Qi. The Five Elemental Phases are an expansion of that concept and they further refine our understanding of Qi. If the yin-yang concept looks at what the road of Qi is made of, then the Five Elements concept looks at the nature of that road—where it rises to cross the mountains and where it plunges to cross the valley floor.

THE FIVE ELEMENTS

Firstly, it is important to note that the Five Elements theory is not a Chinese version of the western Four Elements theory with an extra element thrown in! The only similarity between the two theories is the use of the word element and on closer inspection even this proves to be an illusion.

As the traditional Chinese studied yin and yang in greater and greater depth they found that these two terms became inadequate in the same way that the term 'a day' may refer to 24 hours but does not distinguish between morning, afternoon, evening and night.

In the first instance it is easy to see that 'day' is yang to 'night' which is yin. Within 'day' and 'night' though it is perhaps not as easy to see whether 'morning' is yin or yang to 'afternoon' and whether 'evening' is yin or yang to 'night'. Nevertheless, morning, afternoon, evening and night all have a cyclical similarity to the progression from spring to summer, autumn and winter, or from childhood to adolescence, maturity and old age.

To understand why this is so let us return to the analogy of electricity. When we move from direct current to alternating current we find that we can measure the total current or voltage and the pulse or cycle of the current as it flows back and forth. Qi has its own pulse which can be represented in mathematical form.

In terms of the yin-yang concept, when the graph is rising it is in its yang phase, and when it is falling it is in its yin phase. However, from a mathematical viewpoint, there are not two inflexion points; there are four—the two we expect to see at the top and bottom of the pulse but also two additional ones halfway up (or halfway down) the pulse. The inflection points are important mathematically because they represent the point at which the nature of the graph changes. Thus:

- • - FROM THE INFLEXION POINT AT THE BOTTOM OF THE PULSE THE LINE RISES FASTER AND FASTER UNTIL IT IS VERTICAL.
- • - FROM THE INFLEXION POINT HALFWAY UP THE PULSE THE LINE BEGINS TO RISE MORE SLOWLY UNTIL IT IS MOMENTARILY HORIZONTAL AT THE TOP OF THE PULSE.
- • - FROM THE INFLEXION POINT AT THE TOP OF THE PULSE THE LINE BEGINS TO DROP AWAY FASTER AND FASTER UNTIL AT THE INFLEXION POINT HALFWAY DOWN THE PULSE IT IS ONCE AGAIN VERTICAL.
- • - FROM THE INFLEXION POINT HALFWAY DOWN THE PULSE THE RATE OF DESCENT BEGINS TO SLOW UNTIL FINALLY AT THE LOWER INFLEXION POINT IT IS ONCE AGAIN MOMENTARILY HORIZONTAL.

Wouldn't it be interesting if the pulse that underlay the day or the seasons or the business cycle or the lifecycle reflected the same types of changes? The Chinese refer to the first part of the pulse as the Wood Phase. This period is equated with spring, when there is a burst of growth that becomes more and more active as we move towards the next phase. The second part of the pulse is called the Fire Phase. At this point the energy is at its strongest but it is reaching its peak. This period is equated with summer. The third part of the pulse is called the Metal Phase. (Metal symbolises that which is distilled or refined, such as metal and other precious stones taken from a rocky ore.) You might call it the 'harvest season'. This period is equated with autumn. The fourth part of the pulse is called the Water Phase. At this time the energy is at its most quiescent but it is also a time of preparation for renewal. This period is equated with winter.

'What happened to the fifth elemental phase?' I hear you say. The fifth element is called the Earth element and it is regarded as the 'centralising element'. If you took out the centralising Earth element there would be no pulse or cycle of Qi. The Earth element should be considered an 'inward' direction—one that is somehow part of all directions—north, south, east and west. If you are going to make any sense of the Ba Kua or the *I Ching* you must first understand the special, centralising, inward drawing power of the Earth phase.

I remain fascinated by the fact that the Chinese emperor's throne was always placed on a square symbolising Earth under a curved surface (not a representation of a two-dimensional circle) representing 'heaven'. Have we missed something through paper's inability to represent the third dimension? Were the ancient Chinese philosophers trying to tell us that we must account for additional dimensions when talking about heaven?

ANIMAL SYMBOLS OF THE FIVE ELEMENTS

Each of the five elemental phases is associated with a real or mythical animal:

WOOD	GREEN DRAGON
FIRE	RED PHOENIX
METAL	WHITE TIGER
WATER	BLACK TURTLE
EARTH	YELLOW SNAKE

These associations are intended to convey something of the nature of each phase in the energy cycle. You will need to understand what these animals symbolise to the Chinese if you are to make sense of what the Chinese are saying about the nature of these energy phases.

GREEN DRAGON—WHITE TIGER

In Chinese tradition dragons are not monstrous, fire-breathing reptiles that go around devouring young maidens and testing would-be heroes. Rather they symbolise a primal, powerful, beneficent aspect of natural energy—a source of energy which, if tapped into, can help promote and sustain growth and development. Dragons are yin creatures as they symbolise a gathering of energy or Qi that may then be used for other purposes. The 'dragon' symbol reinforces the 'wood' symbol, as both relate to growth and support. The green colour obviously reinforces the wood symbol but the colour is also seen as regenerative and is associated with improving health. It is a restful colour.

The Green Dragon is paired with the White Tiger, which represents the metal phase of energy. The colour white is seen as a purifying, cleansing colour that reinforces the concept of the pure metal separating from the impure ore. In Chinese terms the Tiger is powerful but dangerous—almost literally a double-edged sword.

The White Tiger is yang to the Green Dragon. It is not unusual to see Chinese artworks depicting the battle or conflict between the Tiger and Dragon. This battle symbolises the eternal conflict between the yin and yang aspects of the universe. The conflict simultaneously contains elements of opposition, transformation and complementation, and is often seen as a representation of the eternal battle of the sexes. Just as this conflict drives the renewal and regeneration of the human race within the human sexual arena, on a cosmic scale it drives the renewal and regeneration of the universe itself.

RED PHOENIX—BLACK TURTLE

While the Black Turtle is yin in relation to the Red Phoenix, the Phoenix and Turtle are nowhere near as strong a symbol of the eternal yin-yang conflict. The Turtle represents the consolidating aspect of yin (yin becoming more yin) as opposed to the Green Dragon, which represents its transforming aspect (yin becoming yang). This is captured perfectly on our graph, for while the Dragon and the Turtle phases of energy are both at the lower (or yin) part of the energy wave, the Dragon is rising (transforming) while the Turtle is falling (consolidating). Likewise, the Red Phoenix and White Tiger are both in the yang part of the energy wave but the Red Phoenix is yang becoming more yang (consolidating) while the White Tiger is yang becoming yin (transforming). The conflict between the transformative aspects of yin and yang is more significant than the consolidative aspects because this is where change and renewal occurs. Because these energy phases are consolidating they do not reach out to cause a meeting between yin and yang and this axis is therefore less important.

The colour red symbolises activity, energy, movement, and that which is consuming. The association with the bird is particularly strong. The colour black has often been associated with that which is hidden, secret, and out of sight—it is characteristic of shelled animals such as turtles and tortoises to retreat rather than oppose.

THE LONELY YELLOW SNAKE

The poor old Snake seems to be almost invisible in any western review of the five elements. Perhaps this is because the Snake is held in such low esteem in the west—a cold, cruel dangerous reptile who led us down the garden path and out of Eden! Also, it seems that the Snake is not partnered with any of the other animal symbols—it is an isolated outcast and what are we supposed to make of that?

Curiously enough, while the Chinese have no great love for the snake family they associate the symbolic snake with knowledge, wisdom and 'a tying together of all things'. In one sense the Snake is yin in respect to all the other elements. It is that which lies at the core—the Earth Element. Yellow of course is a very symbolic colour—the colour of the sun and of gold. It is another purifying colour but unlike white, which purifies in a subtracting way, yellow cleanses in an enriching way.

Let's look at some practical applications of the five elements that can be carried out using the concepts of the Stimulatory and Inhibitory energy cycles.

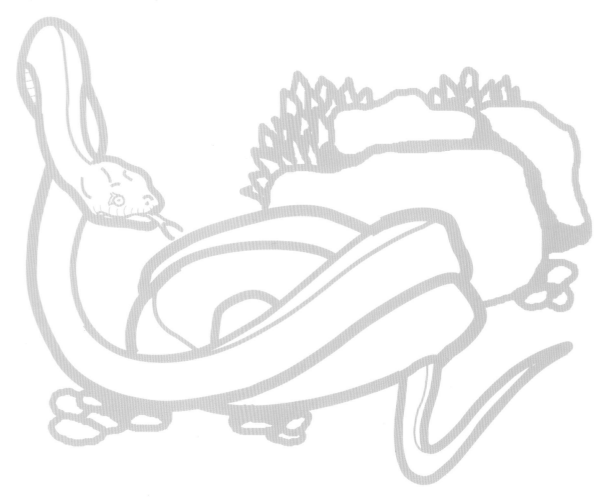

CREATIVE AND CONTROLLING ENERGY CYCLES

These cycles are called various different names, but the most common is the 'Creative' and 'Destructive' energy cycles. While they are indeed opposites, I dislike using the term 'Destructive' because the word generates the idea that some elements need to be kept separate.

In fact what these energy cycles really try to tell us is that there are things we can do to push the energy cycle along and things we can do to slow it down. It is not beneficial to us if the energy pulse becomes distorted or gets out of balance. Study of the energy cycles allows us to predict how these distortions might reveal themselves, then balance or correct the energy pulse. All elements must be in a balanced mix of some sort and one part of the energy cycle cannot simply 'go missing'. For instance, organs relating to all five elements are found within my body but just because my kidneys represent the Water element and my heart represents the Fire element I don't consider having one of those organs removed.

Each phase of the energy cycle can also be seen as the source of the next phase. The elements have the following tendencies towards transformation:

WOOD IS THE SOURCE OF FIRE
FIRE IS THE SOURCE OF EARTH
EARTH IS THE SOURCE OF METAL
METAL IS THE SOURCE OF WATER
WATER IS THE SOURCE OF WOOD,

But in the controlling cycle:

WOOD CONTROLS EARTH
EARTH CONTROLS WATER
WATER CONTROLS FIRE
FIRE CONTROLS METAL
METAL CONTROLS WOOD

What we have seen so far is that yin-yang interactions are responsible for various energy pulses that beat below the surface of our universe in a similar manner to the way that our heart beats within our body. When the energy pulse is in a particular part of its cycle we can predict certain effects which may then be enhanced or inhibited. The theory presented so far provides the basis for predicting the effect of energetic changes using Nutritional Qigong, Environmental Qigong and many other Qigongs (see chapter five). The theory is always the same despite the fact that the practical methodology of Qigongs may vary.

THE BA KUA—QI AND THE HARMONY OF THE EIGHT DIRECTIONS AND BEYOND

Yin and yang can be represented by one broken and one unbroken line.

When represented thus we have the one possibility—yin and yang. If we use two lines then we have four possibilities.

These equate to the form of lesser and greater yang, and lesser and greater yin.

If we have three lines (a trigram) we then have eight possible reflections of the various stages of yin and yang. These appear below along with their Chinese name.

CHIEN   TUI   LI   CHEN

SUN   KAN   KEN   KUN

Together these eight trigrams make up the Ba Kua, which translates as 'The Eight Directions'. A legend says that this concept was revealed to Fu Hsi, the first of the three founding emperors, by a mythical creature that was half horse (yang) and half dragon (yin), and that had the eight trigrams on its back. After 5000 years of study the Chinese still do not consider that they fully understand the symbolic and mystical meanings contained within these symbols.

The *I Ching*, the world's oldest philosophical treatise, is built on the 64 hexagrams that can be made from a 6 line expansion of the trigram known as the Kua. Note that every hexagram consists of two of the eight trigrams—it is just the combination of the trigrams that changes.

Each trigram relates to a direction on Earth when orientated against the Earth's magnetic lines of force. From the

Each trigram relates to a direction on Earth when orientated against the Earth's magnetic lines of force. From the very beginning each trigram represented the nature of Qi energy so in this sense the whole theory was contained within the original trigrams in the same way that you might say all mathematical theory is contained within the concept of numbers even though we keep expanding our mathematical knowledge. The interpretation of the theory and the relation of the hexagrams to practical life was explored over millenia. The I Ching contains commentaries which are guides to interpreting the hexagrams.

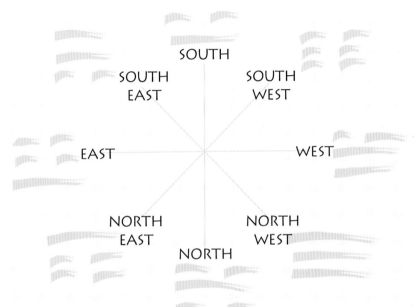

If you simply regard the symbols as 'labels' you will become confused by the fact that the labels can change. If you understand that we are still talking about yin and yang, but in finer permutations, then you will see that we are talking about the direction of energy movements and the nature of the Qi pulse. If you still feel somewhat confused there are two sources of solace.

The first is the words of Kung Fu Tze who reputedly said that even if he had another fifty years to devote to the study of the trigrams he doubted he would obtain a full understanding of their meaning. Two and a half thousand years later we can only agree.

Secondly, as modern science delves into the nature of the universe we are being treated to principles such as the 'Heisenberg Uncertainty Principle', which implies that full knowledge of some aspects of the universe is simply precluded by the nature of the universe. Time dilations, black holes, the ability of subatomic particles to 'know' what related particles are doing half a universe away and the ability of light to be both particle or wave but not both at the same time might persuade us that the nature of the universe is as mysterious as it ever was. Only the boundaries have changed.

With an understanding of the principles raised in this section you will be ready to begin applying these principles through the art of Qigong.

CHAPTER THREE

THE ENERGETIC

BODY

Ask a person who has been brought up in the western tradition,
'What does the body contain?' and they will probably reel off a list that
includes things such as bones, muscles, nerves, cartilage, etc. Now and then you
may find someone who also thinks in terms of 'systems'; the nervous system, immune
system, digestive system, reproductive system, circulatory system, etc. These responses
reflect our cultural preoccupation with the physical. Ask the same question of a person brought
up in the traditional Chinese culture and you will get a quite different answer, with lists of such things
as: Shen Qi, Ren Qi, Wei Qi, Jieng Qi (which all reflect the prime energy fields of the body) or Lung
Qi, Heart Qi, Kidney Qi, Liver Qi, etc (which reflect the energy systems of the body). You may even find
strange concepts such as the three burners or the Jing Lo included. All of these have one thing in common:
they describe various things about the energy of the body.
When we begin to see the body in terms of energy, it is much easier to understand how the subtle energies
around us can influence our body. Now we can focus on such energies as the energy of the physical
environment, the energy of the seasons and the energy of our friends and acquaintances. With this approach,
effects that may simply be dismissed by the term 'placebo effect' in the west can be better understood, for it
is easier to accept that one form of energy can affect another than it is to accept the idea that energy affects
matter or matter systems. Though we can take out the physical heart and look at it, we cannot take out the
energetic heart without changing it, because it is an inseparable part of the body's energetic systems. We
begin then to understand that health is about the whole body, not its component parts. The first
message of the energetic body is be holistic—involve the physical, the mental, the emotional and the
spiritual. The second message is to stop thinking of our body as separate from its surroundings.
Rather, our bodies represent a temporary whirlpool in a river of energy. There is no doubt
that the whirlpool is there but can you separate it from the river? Will not the form and
power of the whirlpool be totally dependent on the nature of the river as we are
dependent on the river of energy that surrounds us?

THE IMPORTANCE OF THE ENERGETIC LANDSCAPE OF THE BODY

Whether you are practising Nei Dan (internal) Qigong or Wei Dan (external) Qigong, the objective is to effect changes on human beings. You might, for instance, think of Nei Dan Qigong as similar to carrying out those processes involved in the selection and construction of a house that included making sure that:

- YOU HAVE THE RIGHT NUMBER OF ROOMS FOR YOUR NEEDS
- THE ELECTRICAL AND PLUMBING SYSTEM IS APPROPRIATE
- THE HEIGHT AND SIZE OF THE ROOMS IS CORRECT.

Wei Dan Qigong on the other hand would be more involved with ensuring that:

- THE HOUSE IS ON THE CORRECT SITE
- THE HOUSE HAS THE CORRECT ASPECT
- APPROPRIATE TRANSPORT AND NEIGHBOURHOOD FACILITIES ARE AVAILABLE
- THE CONSTRUCTION MATERIALS ARE OF GOOD QUALITY.

Both classes of decisions would require that you know something about the inhabitants of the house—how many there are, their age, and any special needs that they might have. In the same way, you need to know about the energy systems residing within your body if you are to successfully practise Nei Dan or Wei Dan Qigong.

Although our focus in this chapter is on human Qigong, note that a Qigong can be developed for any energy system, whether it belongs to another living creature or an inanimate one such as a business, a society or a culture.

GETTING TO KNOW THE ENERGETIC LANDSCAPE OF THE BODY

No-one is surprised to find that the physical body is an incredibly complex system. Billions of cells organise themselves into tissues, organs and systems that operate through complex chemical and electro-chemical reactions. The physical body is so complex that medical specialists spend a lifetime attempting to understand just one of its component parts. This does not mean that the average person cannot obtain a working knowledge of the physical body with the application of a relatively small effort.

The same situation exists with the energetic body. It too is complex and people spend years attempting to master various related applications such as acupuncture, Qi meditation, Qi exercise and so forth. Do not be daunted by this—it is probably easier to obtain a working knowledge and practical understanding of the energetic body than the physical.

In previous sections of this book we have used electricity as an analogy for Qi and I am going to draw on it again to explain another two aspects of Qi: Qi currents and Qi fields.

We know that electricity flows as a current along a wire and that the purpose of the wire is to provide a path of least resistance. Just as water always seeks the lowest path, electricity seeks out the line of lowest resistance. Ren Qi flows like an electric current through the body. While there is no physical 'wire' it is interesting that traditional acu points are located in areas of low electro potential.

But many of us are not aware that this flow of electric current also creates an electric field that extends outwards from the direction of flow of the current. It is simply not possible to have current flow without electrical fields and vice versa. And just as electric currents develop electric fields, these fields create or impact on electric currents.

So Qi also exists as fields and current flows and, again, these are mutually dependent. The physical body concept often deems our mind and emotions an optional by-product of our physical brain and chemistry. But when seen as part of the energetic body, the mind and the emotions are recognised as much more integral components of the universe as a whole.

To build our practical knowledge of the energetic body and better understand its features and landscape we need to learn about the Three Treasures, the Tan Tien, the Jing Lo system, the Zhang Fu organs and the Ren Qi transformation system.

SAN JIAO—THE THREE TREASURES

The Chinese use the term 'San Jiao' or 'The Three Treasures' to denote the most valuable and influential items within a group of items. From a cultural viewpoint, the San Jiao are Taoism, Buddhism and Confucianism. When the Chinese look at Qi from a human perspective, the most important concepts are Jieng (Essence) Qi, Ren (Human) Qi and Shen (Spirit) Qi.

THE FIRST TREASURE—JIENG QI

Jieng Qi is perhaps the most difficult 'energetic' concept to grasp. It is usually described as 'an essence' or 'the essential energy'. Using our previous analogy of electricity, Jieng Qi is more like a field than a current. Consider a magnet, which has lines of force that can be shown by sprinkling iron filings on a piece of paper and placing the magnet under the paper. Together these 'lines of force' make up a 'magnetic field'. We can test the strength of this field by seeing how large a piece of iron it can move or the amount of energy we must expend to bring the like poles of two magnets together, but what is the essence of this field? From where does it derive its strength and power? From the alignment of iron atoms the magnet contains. If we damage the magnet by dropping it repeatedly we gradually weaken and destroy its magnetic field as the atoms of the magnet lose their alignment. The 'Jieng' of the magnet is found in the pattern of its atoms.

Similarly, the essence or 'Jieng' of a human may well be contained within their 'atomic pattern', the blueprint held within the DNA or genetic material of the cell. It has been shown that single cells hold the entire prenatal pattern of the body. Hormones (with which Jieng is often associated) play an important mediating role in ensuring that the cells of the body hold a particular reflection of that pattern at any point in time. When hormones are lost or exhausted the integrated pattern of function begins to deteriorate. I suspect that as we learn more about the mechanisms that direct growth from a single cell to a complex differentiated system such as our body, our concept of Jieng will become clearer.

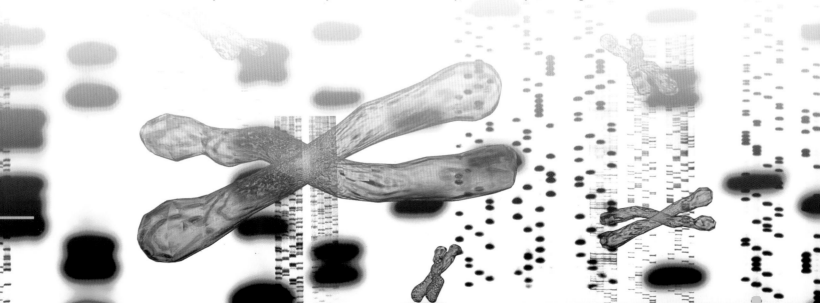

THE SECOND TREASURE—REN QI

Ren Qi literally means Human Qi but is often abbreviated to Qi because all the Qigongs in this area were designed to work with human beings and the term Ren Qi became redundant. I shall however continue to use the term for clarity as this book looks at more than just Human Qi. Ren Qi can be further divided into two major types: Yuan Qi (Prenatal Qi) and Jen Qi (Postnatal Qi).

YUAN QI

Yuan Qi is the Qi that we are born with. It is stored within the adrenal glands of both sexes and in the testes of the male and the ovaries of the female (where it will then provide the Yuan Qi of the next generation). There is some disagreement about whether or not the Prenatal Qi we get at the beginning of our life is all we get. Some see the ageing process as the physical reflection of diminishing Qi. The idea is that we should be living off our 'Postnatal Qi' (see Jen Qi, below).

I find it helpful to think of Yuan Qi as the charge on a car battery. The battery must hold a sufficient charge to start the engine or the car is effectively dead. When the engine is running the generator recharges the battery, but if that charge is not equivalent to the charge being used by the battery, the battery will gradually run down and the engine will not be able to start.

We previously compared Jieng Qi to the genetic pattern of DNA, noting that the 'better' the DNA, the better the potential for a healthy physical constitution. How does Yuan Qi differ from this? It is like the difference between conception and birth. We may be conceived with potentially strong Jieng Qi, but what happens during pregnancy determines our Yuan Qi. Any damaging energies the foetus is exposed to will reduce the Yuan Qi that it is born with.

JEN QI

Jen Qi is the energy that we obtain from our environment. In looking at Nei Dan (internal) Qigong in chapter four we focus on food and air because our internal systems (such as the digestive system and the respiratory system) specifically process and transform Jen Chi energy.

When you think about it, all our senses deal with incoming energy to our body. The light that falls on our eyes falls on our bodies. The sound that causes the vibration of the cilia within the ear vibrates every cell of our bodies. Our sense of hot and cold tells us the nature of the energy flow from the environment and so on. These aspects of Qi are more often dealt with in Wei Dan Qigong, particularly in such skills as Feng Shui, but they are certainly a source of energy whose effects must be taken into account.

Jen Qi has two functions within the body: first as Ying Qi or 'nourishing Qi' and second as Wei Qi or 'defensive Qi'. These may be seen as the 'current' and 'field' aspects of Jen Qi.

THE THIRD TREASURE—SHEN QI

Shen Qi is the energy that sustains the spiritual and intellectual mind. This includes refined emotions and qualities such as wisdom, compassion, love and empathy. I use the term 'refined' because I don't want you to think that emotions are bad and one must aim to become 'emotionless'.

There are only three things that you can do with emotions—express them, repress them or transform them. We know the negative consequences that can arise from the expression of our raw emotions and the even worse things that can happen if they are repressed. The Qigong adherent seeks to transform or refine his or her emotions. The emotionless person cannot be loving, compassionate or empathetic and rarely has much in the way of wisdom, for it is the transformed energy of the raw emotions that powers these things.

The ultimate goal of the energy transformation process in the body is harmonisation of the Shen.

THE THREE TAN TIEN

The term 'Tan Tien' translates as 'the Elixir Field'. In this context 'field' refers to the type of field that one might find in the countryside, though it is also suggestive of the 'energetic field' element.

Most people initially have a concept of the body's energy system that involves Qi flowing through a series of channels or meridians, much as water flows through a plumbing system. This is a good start but it overlooks the fact that the body's 'plumbing system' itself is energetic in nature and interacts with the Ren Qi. The three Tan Tien each store subtly different Qi and each organ system subtly changes the Qi. For example, the Ren Qi that flows within the lung meridian is subtly different from the Ren Qi that flows within the other meridians.

It is perhaps better to think of Ren Qi as being like water in the natural water cycle. At different stages of this cycle it may be the salty water of the ocean, evaporated moisture condensing as clouds, precipitation in the form of rain, snow or hail, mineralised groundwater erupting as a geyser or a spring generating a mountain stream. The changes that water goes through in the water cycle are in many ways more strange than the changes that Ren Qi goes through as it flows through the landscape of the body.

If the currents of Qi can change and transform it follows that the Qi fields associated with those currents can transform too. This is in fact what the concept of the three Tan Tien suggests.

While the three Tan Tien have no 'physical structures' associated with them they do have special properties or attributes. Can we find a parallel to such a situation in nature? Well, we cheerfully talk about the 'poles' of a magnetic field without ever thinking that all we are doing is ascribing particular attributes to the nature of a magnetic field at one point in space. The 'pole' is not something separate from the magnetic field; it is an attribute of it. In the same way we should think of the three Tan Tien as being attributes of the body's energetic field—though in this case there are three rather than two to consider. The Three Tan Tien are:

- • - SHANG DAN TIEN (UPPER TAN TIEN). LOCATED IN THE FRONT UPPER PART OF THE HEAD, THIS TAN TIEN IS ASSOCIATED WITH THE PINEAL AND PITUITARY GLANDS. SHANG DAN TIEN IS THE RESIDENCE OF REFINED SHEN QI.

- • - JONG DAN TIEN (MIDDLE TAN TIEN). LOCATED AT THE LEVEL OF THE SOLAR PLEXUS, THIS TAN TIEN IS THE RESIDENCE OF THE RAW REN QI THAT RESULTS FROM THE MIXING OF YUAN QI AND JEN QI.

- • - SHIAH DAN TIEN (LOWER TAN TIEN). THIS IS THE AREA OF 'MOVING QI' THAT EXISTS IN FRONT OF AND BETWEEN THE KIDNEYS. SHIAH DAN TIEN'S CHIEF CONNECTION POINT WITH THE SURFACE OF THE BODY IS QI HAI OR THE SEA OF QI POINT, LOCATED ABOUT THREE FINGERWIDTHS BELOW THE NAVEL. THIS TAN TIEN IS THE RESIDENCE OF YUAN QI CONVERTED FROM THE ORIGINAL ESSENCE, YUAN JIENG.

The three Tan Tien are not to be confused with 'the Three burners' (which together compose the 'Triple burner meridian'—refer to the Jing Lo system over the page. The Triple burner meridian deals with the balancing of energy levels in the body, whereas the three Tan Tien deal with the progessive refinement and transformation of Qi.

THE JING LO SYSTEM

The Jing Lo system includes the major system of channels (the Jing) and the networks of smaller channels (the Lo) through which Ying (nourishing) Qi flows. Twelve major channels are associated with organ functions and eight other vessels are associated with storing and balancing Ying Qi. Over 700 Xue ('needle points' or 'acupressure points' which are particularly important for adjusting Ying Qi flows) or pockets or cavities of Qi have been located where these channels run along or close to the surface of the skin.

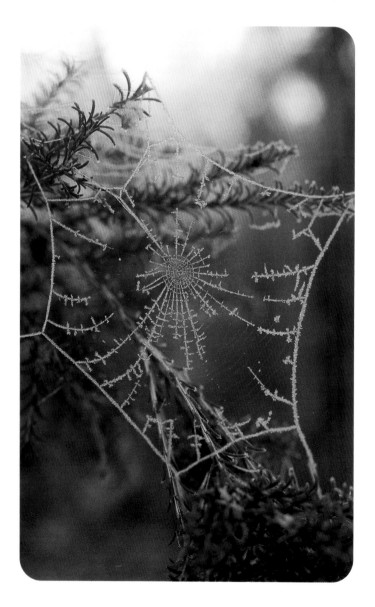

The Jing Lo system is as complex and pervasive as the body's network of nerves or blood vessels. While for practical purposes the focus is often on the major Qi flow channels, these all have their own 'capillary network' that reaches out to every cell in the body. Also, again for practical reasons, the focus tends to be on those parts of the energy channels that are on or close to the surface. It should not be forgotten that the channels connect the internal organs of the body and that these deep channels are potentially much more significant from an energy perspective than their surface extensions. Fortunately they are generally buried deep out of harm's way.

Another useful analogy for the Jing Lo is a spider's web, for any movement or change in one strand (or channel) is felt throughout the entire web.

THE ORGAN MERIDIANS

The term 'organ meridian' is perhaps a little misleading. When we speak of an energy flow being associated with a particular organ it is better to think more in terms of that organ's function than of the physical organ itself. This is because we are talking about energy processes that may not be confined to one particular location.

Do not fall into the trap of thinking that certain organs have a meridian and others don't. Instead, think about it from the perspective that each meridian reflects itself through the organ or organs necessary to carry out that energetic function. Indeed some organ meridians have no 'physical organ' in the western sense—the pericardial sac associated with the 'Heart Protector' meridian is hardly an organ in the western sense of the word, and the 'Triple burner' or 'Three heater' meridian has no identifiable physical manifestation whatsoever.

YIN-YANG PAIRS OF RELATIONSHIPS

THE LUNG MERIDIAN (YIN) / THE LARGE INTESTINE MERIDIAN (YANG)

THE STOMACH MERIDIAN (YANG) / THE SPLEEN MERIDIAN (YIN)

THE HEART MERIDIAN (YIN) / THE SMALL INTESTINE MERIDIAN (YANG)

THE BLADDER MERIDIAN (YANG) / THE KIDNEY MERIDIAN (YIN)

THE PERICARDIUM MERIDIAN (YIN) / THE TRIPLE BURNER MERIDIAN (YANG)

THE GALL BLADDER MERIDIAN (YANG) / THE LIVER MERIDIAN (YIN)

THE DAILY QI CYCLE

Of the twelve organ meridians, six are yang and six are yin. The yang meridians are located on the back and outside surface of the limbs. The yin meridians are located along the front and inside surface of the limbs. Ying Qi flows through the meridians in a particular direction from one meridian to another, completing the entire cycle in 24 hours.

	MOST YANG	MOST YIN
THE HEART MERIDIAN	(11AM–1PM)	(11PM–1AM)
THE SMALL INTESTINE MERIDIAN	(1PM–3PM)	(1AM–3AM)
THE BLADDER MERIDIAN	(3PM–5PM)	(3AM–5AM)
THE KIDNEY MERIDIAN	(5PM–7PM)	(5AM–7AM)
THE PERICARDIUM MERIDIAN	(7PM–9PM)	(7AM–9AM)
THE TRIPLE BURNER MERIDIAN	(9PM–11PM)	(9AM–11AM)
THE GALL BLADDER MERIDIAN	(11PM–1AM)	(11AM–1PM)
THE LIVER MERIDIAN	(1AM–3AM)	(1PM–3PM)
THE LUNG MERIDIAN	(3AM–5AM)	(3PM–5PM)
THE LARGE INTESTINE MERIDIAN	(5AM–7AM)	(5PM–7PM)
THE STOMACH MERIDIAN	(7AM–9AM)	(7PM–9PM)
THE SPLEEN MERIDIAN	(9AM–11AM)	(9PM–11PM)

This indicates the time at which a particular meridian is most active (yang) and least active (yin). Knowing the times a meridian is at its highest and lowest peak of activity is useful in rebalancing the energy of the meridians.

However, a problem with the energy of one meridian does not always have its source in that meridian. An important relationship called the mother/child relationship draws our attention to the fact that the meridian that flows into another nurtures it. If the 'child' meridian is deficient, it may be because the 'mother' meridian is supplying too little energy. The reverse problem may also exist. Meridians also have a husband/wife or paired relationship (see previous page). Interestingly, for the system to work correctly, the relationship must always favour the yang. Since any relationship that favours the yang must ultimately deplete and exhaust, this theory suggests that ageing is a natural process from an energetic viewpoint.

There is also a brother/sister relationship based on meridians belonging to the same 'element'. There are six pairs but only five elements because four meridians are associated with the Fire element: The Heart/Small Intestine and Triple Burner/Pericardium. I also find it interesting that this again suggests a yang imbalance in organic systems.

THE EXTRAORDINARY VESSELS

The word 'vessels' is used instead of meridians here because despite their elongated shape, they store Qi instead of flowing it in a specific direction. Their function is to ensure that the Qi in the meridian system never runs dry or gets dangerously high. As discussed earlier, the traditional Chinese essentially see all illness as a blockage or disruption to the proper flow of Qi. The flows of the extraordinary vessels allow these blockages to be circumvented to some degree.

> Du Mei (Governing vessel—yang)
> Ren Mei (Conception vessel—yin)
> Chong Mei (Thrusting vessel—yang)
> Dei Mei (Belt vessel—yin)
> Yang Chiao Mei (Heel vessel—yang)
> Yin Chiao Mei (Heel vessel—yin)
> Yang Wei Mei (Linking vessel—yang)
> Yin Wei Mei (Linking vessel—yin)

The points at which the vessels cross the paths of the meridians are the points at which the Qi exchange takes place. The Xue that directly influence the energy release of the eight extraordinary vessels are located at these junction points.

These eight vessels are extraordinary as a group, but the first two are also extraordinary within the group. In many ways, the Du Mei is associated with the brain and the Ren Mei with the reproductive organs. These meridians have a special flow direction of Qi, and they are seen as something quite special, above and beyond the organ meridians.

Together Du Mei and Ren Mei make up the 'prime' energy circuit of the body. The Du Mei is linked to the six yang meridians and the Ren Mei to the six yin meridians. Qigong aims to ensure that this 'circuit' is functioning correctly. A number of techniques are used for this, including acupressure and meditation for the 'microcosmic orbit' or lesser heavenly circulation. These are discussed in 'Mindpower Qigong', in chapter five.

In summary, the extraordinary vessels differ from the organ meridians in that they flow in either direction, are like a reservoir of energy that balances the flow of Ying Qi in the other channels, and are not associated with any particular organ.

THE XUE

Along the meridians lie small cavities or pockets of Qi known as Xue. Their position is measured using the body itself as the measuring tool. Thus a person's Qi Hai point is located on the surface of the abdomen, at a point three (of those person's) fingerwidths below the navel.

Traditionally just over 700 Xue points were classified. While most lie on the meridians, a number of special points have no particular relation to any meridian. More recently it was discovered that the ears have some 230 points which do not lie on meridians.

When certain points or sequences of points are pressed or otherwise stimulated they have a very specific effect on the energetics of the body. These points or sequences of points can be used to maintain health and vitality or to correct an energy imbalance. In the west the points are mainly known for their pain relief and anaesthetic qualities but this is a very limited use of their potential.

The energy flow in a Xue can be stimulated through:

- ACUPUNCTURE
- MOXABUSTION (BURNING THE HERB MUGWORT CLOSE TO THE ACUPOINT: MUGWORT IS ESPECIALLY EFFICIENT AT CARRYING HEAT QI INTO THE BODY)
- APPLICATION OF BALMS AND OINTMENTS
- ACUPRESSURE (INCLUDING BIOKINETIC TECHNIQUES)
- MEDITATION.

While acupuncture is the most 'powerful' technique it is also the most invasive and the one that requires the greatest technical skill. Other techniques are listed here in descending order in terms of their invasiveness.

In chapter five we shall look at specific techniques for improving Qi flow through the Xue. Meditating on Qi can be as simple as focusing the mind on a Xue point. This mental focus or attention is sufficient to influence the Qi in the Xue point. It requires very little training and can be practised by anyone.

THE ZHANG FU ORGANS

It should now be clear that the Chinese see form and function as a reflection of the nature of the underlying Qi. The internal organs have form and functions, so inevitably, the Chinese sought to understand the underlying nature of the energy that each organ represents. The system they evolved is known as the Zhang Fu system. It is another important way of understanding the energetic landscape of the body. In the Zhang Fu system the internal organs are divided into 'solid' and 'hollow' categories. Again, this classification system is a way of interpreting and correcting energy imbalances within the body.

Zhang organs are 'solid'. They produce and store energy and are therefore considered yin. The Zhang organs include the heart, liver, kidneys, spleen and lungs. Only the Zhang organs are associated with emotions and the senses, reflecting the nature of their source, yin.

Fu organs are 'hollow'. They regulate and transform energy and are therefore defined as yang. The Fu organs include the stomach, bladder, gall bladder and the large and small intestine. The Fu organs support the same energetic function as the Zhang organ to which they are partnered. Each organ pair has a relationship with one of the Five Elements.

ZHANG	FU	ELEMENT
LIVER	GALL BLADDER	WOOD
HEART	SMALL INTESTINE	FIRE
PERICARDIUM	THREE HEATER	FIRE
LUNGS	LARGE INTESTINE	METAL
KIDNEYS	BLADDER	WATER
SPLEEN	STOMACH	EARTH

There is a group of organs which have both Zhang and Fu characteristics. These include the brain, bones, blood vessels and uterus and are classified as being 'Extra Fu'.

A HANDFUL OF QIS

Ren Qi takes on a number of other names as it performs various functions and actions within the human body. These include:

YING QI

Ying Qi is the current of energy that flows within the Jing Lo system of meridians, channels and their various tributaries throughout the body.

WEI QI

Wei Qi is the defensive energy of the body. It protects us against extremes of climate—not just hot and cold but also dampness and dryness. It is like an energy field that permeates every cell of the body. We know that infection and disease travel as viruses and bacteria and that they are present in our environment all the time, yet it is only every now and then that they succeed and invade us. Should we be surprised if our immune system has an energetic as well as physical component?

Cold feet and viral propagation through the lungs are not related, yet every parent will tell you that if your child has been playing barefoot in a cold, damp environment there is an almost inevitable consequence—a 'cold'. An interesting name in itself.

YI QI

Yi Qi is the energy of the intellectual mind. It includes qualities such as willpower, intellect, memory, analytical and computational ability. In our society the intellectual mind and the emotional mind (see Hsin Qi opposite) are often seen as being in conflict, and this can happen all too easily. The stereotypes of the 'dumb athlete perpetually unable to control their emotions' and the 'cold calculating scientist perpetually unable to find any emotions' are all too familiar. In traditional Chinese terms the intellectual mind and the emotional mind are the two pillars that support the spiritual mind.

HSIN QI

Hsin Qi is the energy that sustains the Heart mind or 'emotional' mind—the raw emotions such as desire, hate, joy, sadness, anger and fear. It is said that the source of Hsin Qi is the Jen Qi we derive from eating and breathing, though I believe that sensory input and our activities also contribute.

Thus the expression in the *Tao Te Ching*:

> THE FIVE COLOURS BLIND THE EYE
> THE FIVE SOUNDS DEAFEN THE EAR
> THE FIVE FLAVOURS DULL THE TASTE
> RACING AND HUNTING MADDENS THE MIND.

The point here is that overindulgence or overstimulation of the senses results in a lack of ability to discriminate both sensually and intellectually. This is not an injunction to see, hear and taste nothing. Nor is it an injunction not to be involved in stimulating activity. As we shall see throughout the rest of this book, the Taoists who held this philosophy had marvellously refined artistic skills such as painting, music and poetry and they turned everyday activities such as writing, exercising and eating into wonderfully sensuous experiences.

The words are a warning that overindulgence in sensory, mental or emotional stimulation can unbalance us energetically.

THE REN QI TRANSFORMATION SYSTEM

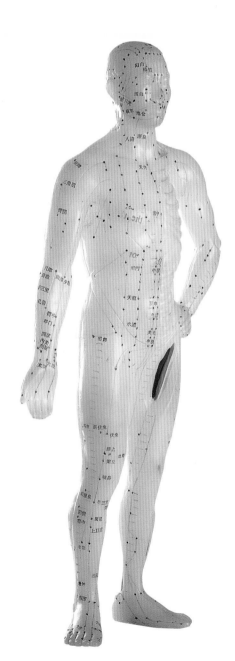

We can now look at how the body transforms Ren (Human) Qi.

Ren Qi is formed from a mixture of prenatal Qi (Yuan Qi) and postnatal Qi (Jen Qi). The prenatal Qi we get from our parents is influenced by the Qi within our environment at the time of conception. The postnatal Qi we obtain from what we eat, breathe and absorb from our environment on a daily basis.

In its 'current aspect' Ren Qi flows through the meridians, where it is called Ying Qi. The nature of this Ying Qi changes as it flows through each organ meridian. Each organ system adds a subtle refinement or transformation of the Ying Qi. These transformations have physical, emotional, mental and spiritual manifestations.

The 'current' of Ying Qi creates various energy 'field aspects'. One of these is Wei Qi, the body's defensive field against pathogens and negative energy. Other field aspects of Ren Qi are centred within the three Tan Tien in progressively more refined forms such as Shen Qi and Yi Qi. When the person is in harmony, Shen Qi and Yi Qi function together as Hsin Qi.

At a very high level, further interactions of Yi Qi and Hsin Qi can result in the generation of Ling Qi, which might be defined as spiritual energy. In Chinese terms all these processes are taking place naturally, but can be improved through Qigong techniques.

THE HUMAN TAO OF QI

In their millennia of experience with Ren Qi the Chinese have discovered many techniques for working with the energy of the human body. The first thing anyone intending to practise the internal arts is told to do is to 'sink the Qi'. The equivalent western expression is to 'centre' oneself. Both expressions are of little use unless you know how to achieve the desired effect.

To 'sink the Qi' one should first establish the correct posture. This involves:

- •. 'The suspended headtop' where we visualise the body hanging down from the crown of the head, like a puppet on a string. The specific acupoint that one visualises the supporting string attached to is the Bai Hui point located at the top of the centre of the head.
- •. 'Sung' which means letting go of all muscular tension not involved in maintaining the posture. Gently releasing the breath will often help achieve this.

When the posture is established, visualise each in-breath going deep into the abdomen (specifically to the Qi Hai acupoint located three of your fingerwidths below the navel). Remember, you are only visualising, not physically forcing your breath to do this. The act of visualising and 'leading' Qi rather than forcing or pushing it is most important. Push Qi and it can end up going anywhere. A traditional Chinese medical expression says 'where the mind goes the Qi flows'.

'Sinking Qi' is important because when Qi is disturbed and dissipated its effects become negative. Let us use the analogy of a farm irrigation system. The water needs to be distributed evenly and gently to the plants. If it is allowed to roar down the channels and overflow in the wrong places it will wash the plants away. Sinking Qi calms and condenses the body's life energy, making it more useful and less destructive. Disturbed Qi disturbs not only the body, but also the mind, emotions and spirit.

'Mian' or 'silk-like movement' is a technique for moving the Qi without disturbing it. When the Chinese drew the silk thread off the silkworm's cocoon they quickly learned that jerky angular movement caused the thread to break. However, if the changes were smooth and even and the movement circular they could change the speed and direction as they drew the thread. The Chinese realised that this concept also applied to Qi and that jerky or angular movements tend to disturb the Qi. One should therefore seek to make one's movements 'silk-like'.

'Sinking the Qi' has a yin effect on the body and every yin activity needs to be balanced by a related yang activity. In this case the complementary activity is 'raising the Shen'. Shen can be translated as 'the spirit of vitality'. It is a refined form of Qi energy that expresses itself as emotions and mood. When the Shen is raised we tend to feel vital, alive and joyous. When the Shen sinks we feel depressed and fatigued.

The 'suspended headtop' technique allows us to relax, sink the Qi and raise the Shen. The Bai Hui point, the point at which we visualise the head being supported by a string, is a strong yang acupoint. Focusing attention on looking forward with the eyes also acts to raise the Shen.

CHAPTER FOUR

NEI DAN

QIGONG

When used to describe a Qigong,
Nei Dan refers to Qigong that works on the Qi
within the body, as opposed to Wei Dan, which refers to work
on Qi that is to enter the human body. This chapter will focus on Nei Dan
Qigongs. Whatever the nature of the Qigong, it is 'work with energy', but first we
must ask ourselves 'work with what purpose?' The answer to this question is happiness.
This is a point often missed by those focused on pursuing physical, mental and spiritual
goals. We do Nei Dan Qigong for health, but why do we want health? Would we want it if we
did not think it was an important part of our happiness? We do Nei Dan Qigong to improve
ourselves mentally and spiritually, but would we want this improvement if it brought misery and
unhappiness? If our goal is to gain physical, mental or spiritual power over others—to be 'the best' or to
'stand out'—we will accept misery and unhappiness to achieve it, but this is not the way of the Tao.
Divorce any goal from the goal of happiness and you will find that your goal is a goal of the ego. Do not
confuse happiness with pleasure. Happiness brings pleasure, but pleasure does not necessarily bring happiness.
What is happiness? Look for inner peace, serenity, and tranquility, keep your sense of wonder and humour, and
you will find it. Perhaps the *Tao Te Ching* says it best:

EMPTY YOURSELF AND BE AT PEACE,

FOR ALL THINGS HAVE THEIR BEGINNING IN ABSOLUTE EMPTINESS.

ALL THINGS CHANGE, GROW AND THEN RETURN TO THE SOURCE.

EVERYTHING COMPLETES ITSELF BY RETURNING TO STILLNESS.

THIS IS THE WAY OF NATURE.

THE WAY OF NATURE IS CONSTANT.

BEING CONSTANT BRINGS YOU INSIGHT.

HAVING INSIGHT YOU WILL GAIN COMPASSION.

GAINING COMPASSION YOU WILL ACT AS AN ANCIENT SAGE.

ACTING AS AN ANCIENT SAGE YOU WILL BE
AT ONE WITH THE TAO.

BEING AT ONE WITH THE TAO
IS LIFE WITHOUT END.

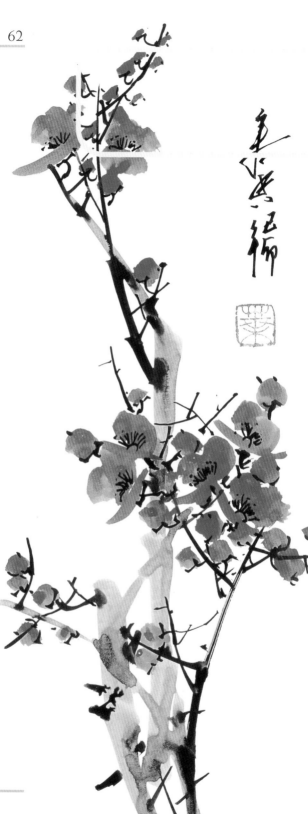

MAY A THOUSAND BLOSSOMS GROW!

Nei Dan Qigongs are those that may be used by a person to work directly on their own Ren Qi (the general name given to Qi in the human body). These Qigongs use posture, movement, breathing and meditation techniques (or some combination thereof) to develop Ren Qi.

There are hundreds (if not thousands) of internal Qigongs. To understand the manner in which they are intended to be used it is necessary to know how these techniques were developed, so we will commence with a general history of Nei Dan Qigong before moving on to look at specific internal Qigongs. It is beyond the scope of any book to explore all the Qigong forms in existence, so I have selected a sample of the Nei Dan Qigongs. These are:

- DAOYIN—TAO-INDUCING EXERCISES
- WU HSIN SI—'FIVE ANIMALS' EXERCISES
- SHAOLIN QIGONG—LOHAN, SINEW-CHANGING AND MARROW-WASHING EXERCISES
- HSING I
- BA KUA GIN—THE EIGHT GOLDEN TREASURES
- TAI CHI
- WEAPON FORMS
- MODERN MIND/BODY/MEDICINE QIGONG

Many books have been written on each of these Qigongs. This book is not a teaching manual for any of these forms—it simply aims to explore the principles and objectives of each.

THE HISTORY OF NEI DAN QIGONG

DANCERS AND BOOK BURNERS

The origins of Qigong are lost in the mists of time. The Yellow Emperor, Huang Di (2697–2597BCE), is usually credited with the development of the Qigong art (along with many other things such as the introduction of coinage and archery). Huang Di is also attributed with authorship of the *Huang Di Nei Ching Su Wen*—The Yellow Emperor's classic treatise of internal medicine. This book is believed to be the first medical book in human history. Traditional Chinese medicine is built on the theory it expounds.

One of the legends about Huang Di is that he was responsible for the first government-sponsored health maintenance program. This was a series of specially designed 'dances' that the population was required to perform for the specific purpose of maintaining health.

Huang Di observed his environment closely and noticed that after floods (which were quite frequent, as his capital was built on the banks of the Yellow River) water lay still on the land and stagnated, the landscape became polluted and foul-smelling and much disease followed. Even then a philosophy was emerging that saw mankind as a smaller reflection of the natural world that surrounded him. Drawing on this philosophy, Huang Di concluded that if sickness resulted from the non-movement or stagnation of water, then sickness would also result in human beings if they did not move about sufficiently. The purpose of these 'health dances' was to maintain the 'internal flow', to prevent disease and maintain health. I do not think there is a better definition of Qigong, so I am happy to credit these 'dances' as the first Qigong forms rather than dance forms or physical exercise forms. The dances were not merely attempts to build muscle, improve stamina or develop breathing or blood circulation (though they would have had these secondary benefits too).

The structure and content of these original dances have been lost and we have no way of knowing what elements of them—if any—have been incorporated into the Qigongs we have today.

What we know about Qigong in the period from the Yellow Emperor to the Qin Dynasty (221BCE) is largely limited to findings from archaeological diggings. The reason for this is that Shang Di, the 'First Emperor' of the Qin Dynasty, was an authoritarian 'book burner' who strictly controlled his inhabitants' access to reading matter and ordered all books other than a limited selection burned. Only a limited number of books survived. The wealth of knowledge and records lost from almost 3000 years of continuous civilisation was incalculable and a major catastrophe for world culture—we are left picking through tombs to glean little pieces of knowledge here and there.

After the Shang Dynasty, China then went through a period very similar to the feudal age that was to arrive in Europe 1000 years later. This was the period of the Chou Dynasty and it lasted for more than 1000 years. Just as the end of the feudal age in Europe saw a great renaissance in learning, art and literature, the disintegration of the Chou Dynasty brought about a period of great intellectual brilliance. Almost every daily activity was affected by the thoughts of these thinkers, and the practice of Qigong and health arts were no exception. (Curiously, across the world in Greece and India a similar flowering of thought and art was taking place at roughly the same time.) In China, the names Kung Fu Tze (Confucius), Lao Tse (author of the *Tao Te Ching*), Mo Ti, Mencius and Chuang Tze are still revered as the profound philosophical thinkers who developed the patterns for philosophical thought that are pursued even to this day.

It was in this period that Daoyin Qigong came to prominence. This art laid the foundation for all future Qigongs, creating a synthesis of physical movement, posture, breathing and meditation techniques, acupressure and acumassage techniques. Daoyin is still practised as a sophisticated and enjoyable Qigong form.

The Han Dynasty marked the next 'great step forward' in Chinese health science. Physicians such as Hua Toe reanalysed the Daoyin, looking to strengthen its balancing effect on the mind and emotions. One result was the creation of the 'Five animal frolics', in which not only the body but also the mind itself must hold the 'spirit' or 'character' of the animal being imitated.

THE SHAOLIN TEMPLE

Following the collapse of the Han Dynasty, traditional Chinese culture continued to flower under the Sui, Tang and Sung dynasties. (This period lasted for almost seven centuries and could perhaps be regarded as the pinnacle of traditional Chinese civilisation.) Throughout these eras there was much contact with the outside world. Many Buddhist monks came from India to promote Buddhism, which subsequently flourished within China. One of the Buddhist monasteries established was the Shaolin Temple, which was destined to become known throughout the world as the birthplace of martial arts.

The most notable abbot of the Shaolin Temple was Bodidharma. He formulated training methods based on a synthesis of physical exercise, martial arts and meditation techniques that were so successful that they became known throughout the world as the Shaolin Forms. (He also formulated a form of Buddhism that was known as 'Chan' in China and 'Zen' in Japan.)

The Shaolin's prestige was so great that it virtually became a university of physical and mental training techniques, and many attended the temple simply to gain this knowledge and discipline. One such person was a Taoist Master, Chan San Feng. While passing through all the training disciplines and attaining the rank of a Shaolin master, Chan San Feng became dissatisfied with the Shaolin forms because they did not express the principles of the Tao. Retreating to the Wu Dang mountains he blended 'hard' Shaolin and 'soft' Taoist traditions, thereby evolving Tai Chi Chuan. Other 'internal' forms that better expressed the Chinese philosophical and health approach also emerged including Hsing I (Mind Boxing, see page 82) and Ba Kua (The eight directions). These, together with Tai Chi Chuan, were to become the three key internal martial arts of China.

With the fall of the Sung Dynasty to Genghis Khan's Mongol Empire, Chinese culture turned inwards and the impetus of the traditional Chinese civilisation was lost. Even when the Chinese re-established control over their own country under the Ming Empire this dynasty focused on the glories of the past rather than the opportunities of the future. Closed to outside contact and fearful of change, the Chinese civilisation that had been centuries ahead of the rest of the world now slipped behind. This brought about the very calamities they had feared: further invasion, this time by the Manchu (a foreign dynasty, not a Han Dynasty). This dynasty was in turn brought down by a combination of internal insurrection and interference by the European powers and invasion by Japan.

In this period of invasion and conflict Qigong became the property of the Triads and other secret societies, and its martial aspects were emphasised (for the overthrow of various oppressors). The Nationalist government that arose in place of the Manchu dynasty did little to re-establish the traditional place of Qigong, and even attempted to ban traditional Chinese medicine. When the Communist party came to power it seemed that they were not only ideologically opposed to Qigong but that they had the control and organisational abilities to eliminate Qigong if they wished.

Several things conspired to turn this moment of ultimate threat to Qigong into a renaissance of the Qigong arts. Firstly, the problems in China had caused Chinese people to disperse over large portions of the globe. In a strange environment they placed new value on the traditional aspects of their culture and sought to preserve them. Secondly, the Chinese who had emigrated soon found that their food and culture were fascinating to the western world and a good way of making a living. It was not long before Qigong techniques that had long been the secret of a chosen few were being revealed through the media of new societies whose whole ethos was the complete dissemination of information. A good example of this was Bruce Lee, who, with his Jeet Kun Do martial art fighting techniques, became a hero to millions of would-be martial artists.

In addition to this, once the Communist government had gained control of China and turned its attention to developing the nation, it had to confront the realisation that it would be decades before the medical infrastructure of the country would be able to meet its needs. One solution was the development of large-scale health exercise programs, the idea being that the healthier the population was, the less strain would be imposed on the existing medical infrastructure. Tai Chi and Qigong were found to be the most effective ways of doing this.

DAOYIN—TAO-INDUCING EXERCISES

We know from archaeological evidence that Daoyin exercises date back at least 2200 years. The name is variously translated as 'Tao-inducing', 'Tao-guiding', 'The gentle approach to the way' and 'Guiding and pulling exercise'.

The exercises are seen by the Chinese as the foundation forms from which the other Qigongs developed. Again, their focus is to stimulate the flow of Qi around the body through the use of the following techniques:

- • TENDON AND MUSCLE STRETCHING
- • BREATHING
- • ACUPRESSURE AND ACUMASSAGE
- • VISUALISATION AND MEDITATION

Despite its antiquity, Daoyin is still practised in China as a form in its own right. It is also practised in Japan as Do-in and has also become the basis of many other systems such as Shin-sen Do. Its flavour is best appreciated through the performance of one of its exercises.

The Taoist *Wu Chi Ching* ('Cannon of the Great Void') eloquently sets out the purpose of Daoyin:

TOUGHEN MY SINEWS, HARDEN MY BONES
MAKE MY BLOOD FLOW FREELY
I WILL THEN BE YOUNG FOREVER
IN TOUCH WITH THE REALM OF THE GODS.

While Daoyin exercises tend to work on the entire energy system, they may have specific benefits that make them particularly beneficial for one organ system. The 'Elegant Crane greets the Morning Sun' exercise on the following page is particularly beneficial for the heart. As you raise your arms and heels, breathe in slowly through the nose and focus on bringing the breath deep into your abdomen. Breathe out as you lower your arms and heels.

THE ELEGANT CRANE GREETS THE MORNING SUN

PART ONE

- Stand with your feet shoulder-width apart. Slowly raise your arms in front of your chest to shoulder height, with your palms facing upwards and fingers pointing forwards. As you do this, lift your heels and let the balls of your feet support your weight.

- Rotate your wrists so that your palms face forwards and your fingers point upright. Curl your fingers inwards so that the pads of your fingertips press into the centre of your palms.

- Slowly lower your hands to your sides while gently bringing your heels to the ground and slightly bending your knees, then release your pressed palms.

PART TWO

- Extend both arms by your side then raise them outwards to shoulder height, with palms facing up. As you do this, straighten your knees, lift your heels, turn your head and look to the left.

- Rotate your wrists so that your fingers point upright with your palms facing outwards. Then curl your fingers so that they press into the centre of your palms.

- Lower your hands to your sides and your heels gently to the ground, bending your knees as you turn your head to face forwards again and release your pressed palms.

REPEAT PART ONE.

PART THREE

- •- Extend both arms by your side, then raise them outwards to shoulder height, with palms facing up. As you do this, straighten your knees, lift your heels and turn your head to the right.

- •- Rotate your wrists so that your fingers point upright, with your palms facing outwards. Then curl your fingers so that they press into the centre of your palms.

- •- Lower your hands to your sides and your heels gently to the ground, bending your knees as you turn your head to face forwards again and release your pressed palms.

REPEAT PART ONE.

PART FOUR

- •- Extend both arms downwards and push your hands behind your body to kidney height, with your palms facing backwards and your fingertips pointing downwards. As you do this, straighten your knees, lift your heels and let the balls of your feet support your weight.

- •- Curl your fingers and press them into the centre of your palms.

- •- Lower your hands to your sides while lowering your heels gently to the ground, then release your pressed palms.

REPEAT PART ONE TO FINISH.

HOW THE ELEGANT CRANE CALMS THE HEART

How does this movement help to 'calm' the heart? Firstly, the movement is done with gentle breathing—eventually you should be able to slow the movement so that each full cycle of breath takes about 15 seconds. This is a breathing rate of four breaths per minute; any breathing rate below about eight breaths per minute moves the body into relaxation response which normalises blood pressure and slows the beating of the heart.

There is a strong link between breath rate and heart rate. When we are stressed, the heart muscle often begins to contract before it is fully relaxed. This means less blood is pumped with each beat. From the body's perspective, overall blood flow is increased because of the rapid beating, but in essence the heart is working inefficiently. This movement helps correct that.

The heart is not designed to be solely responsible for pumping the blood around the system. The muscular walls of arteries contract, and veins threaded through muscles have a series of valves so that each time the muscle contracts it can pump the blood back towards the heart.

In this movement the simultaneous muscular movements in the legs and arms, combined with the lifting of the heel, act to reduce the amount of work the heart has to do in the circulation of blood. The rhythmic movement of the muscles also helps release stress-related tension held in muscles. This is most important, because the heart would otherwise have to maintain pressure high enough to force the blood through these areas of congestion. We must also not forget that within the body torso the diaphragm both powers the lungs and circulates blood through its compressive and relaxation phases. The deeper we breathe, the more assistance the lung diaphragm provides to the heart.

The exercise is quite sophisticated from a physical viewpoint—but what about its energetics? The heart meridian runs down through the arms to terminate in the little finger. If you focus on thrusting the little finger forwards with a light twist of the wrist at the end of each raising movement the heart meridian will be straightened and the heart energy will flow more freely.

When the pads of the fingertips press on the centre of the palm they press the Lao Gong point, which can almost be regarded as a 'safety valve' for heart energy. (You will find this point used in most Qigong exercise systems.)

Last but not least, there is that rather quaint name for the movement. While traditional Chinese names for Qigong movements can often seem a little 'wimpy' to the macho western male, the Chinese were well aware that the imagery or visualisation that we had in our mind could have a profound effect on the flow of Qi. (Few westerners who try Japanese samurai techniques get much involved in poetry or flower arranging although these are important training techniques and elements of the movements.) In this instance the visual image of the cranes waking during the morning and stretching their wings and legs in preparation for the day is useful for developing the proper nature of the movement.

WU HSIN SI—FIVE ANIMALS PLAY

Sometimes called Wu Qin Qigong (Five Animals Qigong), this exercise system is credited to a Han Dynasty physician called Hua Toe, who lived in the second century AD. Like all Chinese health arts, it grew and developed over the centuries, and many separate schools of practice developed, some focusing on different benefits that could be obtained from the exercises.

Hua Toe is credited with realising that previous movement systems had only utilised those parts of the mind that were associated with willpower, concentration, memory and analytical focus (the aspects that we would today classify as 'left brain functions'). Hua Toe found that such exercises were helpful to patients with physical problems, but not of great value to patients with emotional and mental problems. He sought to develop an exercise form that would utilise all aspects of the mind, including the functions of imagination, visualisation and creativity.

Hua Toe did not, of course, have the western concept of left brain/right brain thinking, but he did have the concept of the five elements and the understanding that mental and emotional states could cause disharmony and sickness within the body, and vice versa. Because each animal form is related to a particular element, we can draw on the various associations of organs and emotions associated with each element (listed in the table opposite) to understand the particular uses to which each exercise can be put.

ELEMENT	EXERCISE	ZHANG FU	EMOTION	ORGAN
WOOD	TIGER	LIVER	ANGER	GALL BLADDER
FIRE	BIRD	HEART	JOY*	SMALL INTESTINE
				PERICARDIUM AND
				TRIPLE-BURNER
METAL	DEER	LUNGS	SADNESS	LARGE INTESTINE
WATER	MONKEY	KIDNEYS	FEAR	BLADDER
EARTH	BEAR	SPLEEN	PENSIVENESS	STOMACH

In this table, * Joy should be regarded as 'excessive happiness'. The sort of consequence where an event is so 'joyfully disturbing' that it causes cardiac arrest! All the emotional consequences here are negative ones, representing imbalances that need to be fixed.

Wu Hsin Si postures imitate the postures of such animals as the Tiger, Bird, Deer, Monkey and Bear. It is important to realise that the word 'posture' is not limited to physical postures but relates very much to the emotional and mental posture that one associates with these animals. In other words, in one's practice, one seeks to acquire both the physical and spiritual form of the animal. (The word 'spirit' here has no religious connotation.)

When practising the exercises for general health, it is important that all the exercises are done. To focus on doing just one of the animal exercises could create an energy imbalance, unless you are trying to correct a specific energy imbalance that already exists.

You will often find variations in the nature of movements described. The whole point of these exercises is not to follow instructions with your left brain, but rather to catch the spirit of the animal by recalling what you know of the way it moves and trying to capture the feel or spirit of that movement. You have to be reasonably uninhibited—this very state of mind provides much of the value of the movement.

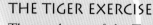

THE TIGER EXERCISE

The attributes of the Tiger are power, strength and mastery. Here it is associated with the Wood Element, but it also carries much of the symbolism of the Dragon as well (in terms of the inherent power of natural forces). The Tiger thus symbolises contained power, just waiting to burst forth.

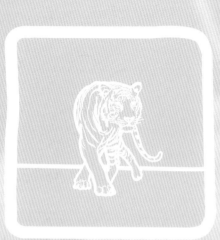

Being associated with the Wood element, the movements have particular benefits for the liver and nervous system. (In Taoist philosophy the liver is the 'root' of the nervous system.)

Tigers have been known to jump two-metre high fences, seize a young calf and jump back over the fence again, carrying the calf in their mouth. This posture is designed to capture such a demonstration of strength.

Breathe in as you assume this posture. Strengthen your spine, looking down while keeping the back of your neck strong, bending your knees and extending your hands forwards and downwards with clawed fingers as though your body is supporting a great weight. Breathe out as you release the posture. Repeat 8 times.

The Tiger exercise is particularly useful in cases of anxiety, hostility and inability to control anger.

THE BIRD EXERCISE

The attributes of the Bird include the ability to soar high into the air above the Earth. In this way the Bird symbolises the spirit and is associated with the Fire element.

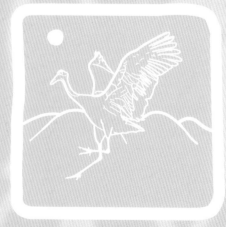

Breathe in as you assume this posture. Raising your hands above your head as though with outstretched wings, keeping your head lifted and eyes alert. Breathe out as you release the posture. Repeat 8 times.

Being associated with the Fire element, the movements have particular benefits for the heart. The Bird exercise is particularly useful in cases of excessive sentimentality and inability to control happiness or joy. It is a centring exercise that creates tranquility and serenity.

THE DEER EXERCISE

The attributes of the Deer are lightness and agility. This animal springs about as though it is weightless and untouched by gravity.

Breathe in as you assume this posture by turning your head as if you are a deer looking to its rear, keeping your hands extended in front with closed fists. Feel light and energetic. Breathe out as you release the posture. Repeat 4 times to each side.

As the Deer is associated with the Metal element, these movements have particular benefits for the lungs. The Deer exercise is particularly useful in cases of excessive sadness and grief, or where we are 'weighed down' by emotion. It is a good exercise to do if you are feeling depressed.

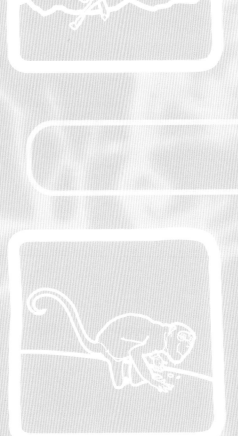

THE MONKEY EXERCISE

The nature of the Monkey is like water: playful and uninhibited. It is not bound by convention and adapts to its surroundings and environment.

Breathe in as you assume the posture of a monkey climbing a tree, with one hand reaching up against the tree to support you and the other reaching out to pick fruit. Raise one foot from the ground and look towards the fruit you are picking. Breathe out and in again as you change the posture so that you are standing on the other foot picking fruit with the other arm. Keep your breathing deep and relaxed, your eyes alert but playful. Repeat 8 times.

As the Monkey is associated with the Water element, these motions are noted for strength-ening the functions of the kidneys and bladder. The monkey exercise is particularly useful in cases of excessive fear and nervousness. It can strengthen willpower and confidence.

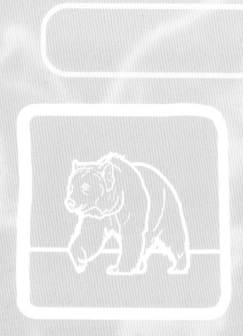

THE BEAR EXERCISE

The attributes of the Bear are weight and mass. Very powerful and balanced, it tends to envelope its prey. It is almost impossible to disturb this animal's centre of gravity. In this the Bear symbolises the Earth element.

Stand with your feet a little wider than shoulder width. Breathe in, keeping a straight spine while allowing your abdomen to relax completely as you tilt forward slightly and let your arms hang loose at your sides, with your knees 'soft'. Feel all the flesh of your body hanging from your skeletal frame. Breathe out as you release the posture. Repeat 8 times.

As the Bear is associated with the Earth element, these movements have particular benefits for the stomach and spleen. The technique is particularly useful for stress, anxiety and irritability. It can strengthen willpower and a sense of centre.

SHAOLIN QIGONG

Of all the tens of thousands of temples that exist in the world, the Shaolin is one of the most well-known. The name is descriptive: 'Shao' is a reference to Shaoshi Mountain, which the temple faces, and 'lin' means 'woods', so the name literally means 'the Shao woods temple'.

The temple is located at the base of Mount Shung (one of the five sacred mountains of China), in the Henan province. When I first went to the Shaolin Temple in the early 1980s, herds of pigs frolicked in the mud of the dirt streets that led to its doors. There were only one or two monks at the temple, most having been dispersed into the countryside during the Cultural Revolution. There seemed little evidence of the legacy that represented Shaolin—even the temple itself seemed unpretentious and unaware of its lineage. It seemed strange to think that Zen and Chan Buddhism and virtually all martial arts from China, Japan, Korea, Taiwan and Vietnam trace their origin to this place. (Even forms created in the west, such as Bruce Lee's Jeet Kun Do, blend forms and styles that originated in this temple.)

Since then the temple has been 'discovered' by the tourist industry. The little peasant town that surrounded the temple now has shiny new facilities, the temple is fully staffed and martial arts training and development are taking place.

The Shaolin Temple has undergone many such changes in fortune over its 1500-year history. Personally, I will always treasure walking in the quiet, deserted, somewhat overgrown courtyards of the Shaolin Temple with nothing to disturb me but the breeze rustling the towering gingko trees studding the temple grounds. These days when I return to the temple and find it full of admiring visitors I cannot help but reflect on a passage from the *Tao Te Ching* :

> LET OTHERS BURDEN THEMSELVES
> WITH THE WEIGHT OF UNNECESSARY THINGS.
> NOTICE HOW THEY STRUGGLE AS TIME GOES BY.
> BECOME CONCERNED WITH COMPLEXITY,
> AND YOU WILL LOSE SIGHT OF SIMPLICITY.
> YOU WILL HAVE TOO MUCH TO REMEMBER,
> AND TOO MUCH TO FORGET.

THE SHAOLIN TRADITION

The Shaolin Temple is often considered 'the birthplace of the martial arts'. This is not to say that martial arts were unknown before the Shaolin Temple, but rather that it was here that martial arts acquired their 'spiritual element' and became a way to improve oneself not just physically and mentally, but spiritually. Here it was realised and accepted that the 'opponent who must be overcome' could be oneself, not necessarily another person.

Without the Shaolin Temple there would have been no Judo, Jujitsu, Karate, Aikido, Tai Chi Chuan, Ba Kua, Wing Chun, Hsing I, Hapkido, Taekwondo and so on. It is simply impossible to imagine where Qigong and oriental martial arts would be without the Shaolin Temple. However, is quite probable that the Shaolin Temple would simply be another unknown temple but for the arrival of that key figure who went by the Indian name Bodhidharma and the Chinese name Ta Mo in about 527CE.

The temple had been established by Batuo, another Indian monk, in 495CE. Little is known about its history before Bodhidharma took over, but apparently when Bodhidharma first cast his eye over the Shaolin Temple he considered the monks to be an indolent lot, completely unfit for the rigors of monastic life. (Bodhidharma was rumoured to have meditated facing a blank rock wall for nine years, so he certainly had mental discipline.) Bodhidharma set about establishing a training regime that would toughen up the monks physically and mentally. His techniques included:

- LOHAN HAND MOVEMENTS
- SINEW-CHANGING EXERCISES
- MARROW-WASHING EXERCISES
- MEDITATION TECHNIQUES SUCH AS THE MICROCOSMIC AND MACROCOSMIC ORBIT.

Gradually these techniques coalesced into a system that became known as the Shaolin Chuan Fau (techniques of the fist). These training methods were arduous and some a little theatrical— including pounding one's hands repeatedly into containers of small iron balls, having tree trunks suspended on ropes swung into one's abdomen like a battering ram and learning to bend spears against one's abdomen or throat. The final test of a Shaolin monk was to pick up a 300-pound (136kg) metal brazier filled with glowing coals. This branded the arms with the Shaolin symbols. It was a final test of strength and the ability to control pain.

However, one must be careful not to confuse these somewhat 'exhibitionist' feats with the real physical and mental discipline that took place within the temple. These feats were not the central element or purpose of the Shaolin forms which were about personal and spiritual development.

The success of the Shaolin Temple resulted in its techniques being adopted within many temples, though none with the prestige of the original Shaolin Temple.

As the basic Shaolin techniques were developed and refined over the centuries they began to be expressed through distinct styles, the five key styles being the Crane, the Snake, the Leopard, the Tiger and the Dragon. These in turn were further developed into such styles as the Preying Mantis, the Eagle, Wing-Chun, Tai Chi, Ba Kua and Hsing I. Shaolin styles were exported to other countries, where they developed into Karate, Aikido, Taekwondo, Hapkido, Judo and so on. Thus while there is a tremendous degree of variation in the appearance of oriental martial arts, when you explore their basic philosophies and principles, you find the Shaolin concepts and techniques at the core of all of them.

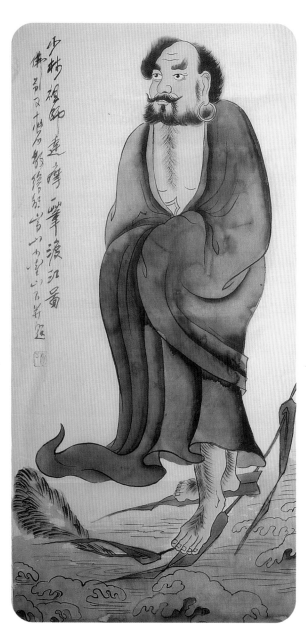

LOHAN HAND MOVEMENTS

Lohan was originally a series of separate postures practised independently rather than as a continuous sequence. It would be reasonable to presume that since Bodhidharma came from India, there is a strong 'yoga' base to Lohan. Various Lohan styles have been preserved within certain families, each claiming that 'their' form is the one that can be traced back to Bodhidharma's original. Because the original form doubtlessly evolved over its millennia-and-a-half of practice, it is unlikely that such disputes will ever be resolved.

While the individual movements included in the Lohan form may vary, the basic principles remain the same. Lohan is a powerful system for generating strength and endurance on a physical, mental and energetic level. Because of its power, proper instruction is essential as injuries at any of these levels can occur when one is first learning the art.

SINEW-CHANGING AND MARROW-WASHING EXERCISES

The individual exercises in these sets are very similar to the Daoyin concept of exercise (see page 67). Whether these exercises were actually created at the Shaolin Temple or it was here that they were put together as a comprehensive health and personal development system will probably always remain a matter of opinion. Both techniques continue to be practised today under variations of the same names, such as the 14 Sinew-changing exercises and the 10 Marrow-washing exercises.

Sinew-changing exercises focus on twisting, turning and stretching movements to develop flexibility and suppleness. In addition to focusing on exercising the bones and sinews, the Sinew-changing and Marrow-washing exercises require particular attention to posture, breathing, mental focus and energy work. In their concern to 'exercise the bones', the Chinese sought to do more than simply increase bone density and reduce bone brittleness. (In the modern world's fight against osteoporosis, the value of weight-bearing exercise has been scientifically proven.) The name Marrow-washing rather than 'Bone-exercising' indicates that the Chinese also understood the importance of bone marrow. Today we know that bone marrow produces many of our red blood cells and our white blood cells, which are very important to our immune system. Marrow-washing exercises not only provide weight-bearing exercise, but incorporate 'Bone-breathing techniques' where one visualises the gathering of Qi into the bones on each in-breath and the condensing of that energy into the bone on the out-breath.

In the west there is often some surprise that the Chinese are apparently unconcerned about the fact that different masters and instructors teach different movements for exercise systems such as Lohan, and Marrow-washing and Sinew-changing exercises. Many westerners are also puzzled about why the same movement may turn up in a number of different exercise systems. This is because the western focus tends to be on the physical aspects of the movement, whereas the Chinese focus is much more on the energetic objectives of an exercise and on the benefits to be achieved. What is important is not that a particular exercise is performed, but that every part of the body is exercised and that the mind is not overlooked in our daily exercise.

YUEH FEI, HSING I AND THE BA KUA GIN

Yueh Fei (960–1127CE) is one of the heroes of the Chinese people, on a par with legendary heroes of the west such as Hercules. Yueh Fei was not just a fighter and strategist; he was also a person of great moral integrity and excelled at many aspects of life. To the Chinese he is the great role model of what one should aim to be. He was the main defence against the incursion of the Mongol hordes—the country collapsed after he was betrayed and poisoned by a corrupt official. In many ways he was a similar figure to Marcus Aurelius of the Roman Empire—the last person of integrity to stand between civilisation and the barbarian hordes that were waiting to destroy it.

Yueh Fei created two martial arts styles: the 'hard' Eagle Claw style and the internal Hsing I style. The latter is of most relevance to this book. He also developed a form of health and strength training for his soldiers known as the Ba Kua Gin (Eight Golden Treasures), a practice that remains popular to this day. Yueh Fei was originally trained by Jou Ton, who had trained and studied at the Shaolin Temple.

HSING I

Hsing I Chuan, generally shortened to Hsing I, is one of the three major internal forms of martial arts, that is it relies on internal energy (Qi) rather than external muscular power. In martial arts terms, Hsing I can be more quickly learned and applied than Tai Chi or Ba Kua. This does not mean that there is less to Hsing I than arts such as Tai Chi, but that the Hsing I student learns the principles *through* the practice of the art, whereas the Tai Chi practitioner learns the principles *to* practise the art.

Hsing I can be translated as 'Mind Form Boxing', but is sometimes called 'Five Elements Boxing'. It is the internal form most closely related in spirit to the Shaolin forms. Unlike Ba Kua and Tai Chi, its nature is linear, so in combat the practitioner constantly moves forward to engage the opponent. When one learns Hsing I, the first objective is to integrate Hsing (form) and I (mind). As this is achieved, one learns how to hide one's own intent within the form but distinguish the opponent's intent within their form so that a pre-emptive strike may be launched. This is what Hsun Tzu meant when he said, 'Begin after the enemy but arrive before him.' Eventually 'mind' and 'form' become spontaneous and there is no conscious form. But how does Hsing I work from a Qigong viewpoint? The Five Elements play an important role as there are five chuan or 'fists', each related to an element. While each chuan is associated with a method of hand strike, it also involves whole body posture, movement technique, breathing, and mental focus. Each 'fist' or 'chuan' is also related through the Five Elements to a particular pair of organ meridians.

WOOD	PENG	(TO CRUSH)	GALL BLADDER/LIVER
FIRE	P'AO	(TO POUND)	HEART/PERICARDIUM/TRIPLE HEATER /SMALL INTESTINE
METAL	P'I	(TO SPLIT)	LUNG/LARGE INTESTINE
WATER	TSUAN	(TO DRILL)	KIDNEY/BLADDER
EARTH	HENG	(TO CROSS)	STOMACH/SPLEEN

The postures associated with each fist align the Qi channels within the body to strengthen the energy flow in the channels related to that element. The nature of the motion and the intention associated with the posture also strengthen the Qi channels associated with that element.

Hsing I also uses animal forms to increase the martial arts techniques available to the practitioner. The Shan Xi style, widely regarded as the most traditional style of Hsing I, uses the Dragon, Tiger, Monkey, Horse, Iguana, Cockerel, Hawk, Snake, Eagle, Bear, Swallow and Phoenix as animal forms.

As in the Wu Hsin Si (Five Animals Play), the objective of each animal form in Hsing I is to capture the spirit or essence of the nature of the particular animal, but the Hsing I practitioner does this while carrying out one of the five chuan techniques. Health benefits similar to those outlined in the Wu Hsin Si can be obtained, with each animal form being associated with a particular Qi flow that works to strengthen the energetic structure of the body.

84

BA KUA

Ba Kua translates as 'the eight directions' or 'the eight changes'. Ba Kua is also the name given to one of the three major soft martial arts. The reason for this association is the circular nature of the art and the palm changes used. Again, the art is said to have emerged from the Taoist temples.

The basis of the movement is circular, with the practitioner walking a circle that is 2–4m in diameter. The stepping pattern uses a lowered stance and a hollowed foot. While travelling around the circle the hands execute a series of movements and the body spins in the reverse direction. A series of spinning, ducking, weaving motions accompany the arm movements.

While the Ba Kua is a very effective martial art technique it also carries with it many philosophical implications. The circle that the Ba Kua Gin practitioner walks represents the circle of the heavens—the Ba Kua.

As with all internal Qigongs, there is a focus on posture (straight back, head held in alignment with sacrum), breathing (diaphragmatic), and the principles of nei-ko (a sense of being internally 'bound' (as though the organs and tissues are being drawn together) and waich'eng (being externally stretched). Another way of explaining this is that movements feel as though they come from the Tan Tien (see page 48).

TAI CHI

'Taijichuan' is the true name for what is popularly known as Tai Chi. 'Tai' means supreme or grand, 'ji' means terminus or ultimate, and 'chuan' means fist or discipline. 'Taijichuan' therefore translates as 'grand ultimate fist'. For various reasons the popular name that the public is familiar with in the west is Tai Chi—I shall use that term in this book.

Chan San Feng was a Taoist who trained at the Shaolin Temple and became a Shaolin master. Discontent with the hard external form of Shaolin, for it sat uneasily with his Taoist training, he retreated to the Purple Cloud monastery in the Wu Dang mountains to contemplate this disharmony. There he either witnessed or had a dream about a fight between a snake and a crane.

The crane (representing the hard Shaolin form) would strike at the snake with its hard beak and deflect the snake's strikes with its wings while hopping about nimbly. The snake (representing the Taoist principles) would coil back as the crane struck and use the energy of its coils to unleash a fluid strike against the crane. The danger the snake represented was the powerful poison buried deep within. The danger the crane represented was its exterior form of beak and claws. Neither opponent could defeat the other.

Chan San Feng saw from this that the ideal form should contain the elements of both snake and crane. The outside body should be soft, fluid and relaxed. One should 'walk like a cat', 'flow like a great river' and 'have the stillness of a mountain'. Internally one should be as 'a cat waiting for a mouse' or 'an eagle about to seize a rabbit'. One should 'soften that which is exterior' and 'strengthen that which is interior'—become iron within cotton wool.

From these concepts Chan San Feng created the 'long chuan' or flowing movement sequence of Tai Chi. Performed slowly, because slowness builds strength, stability and internal tranquility, it removed muscular tension. The body became like water, a placid pool one moment, the next an explosive torrent. Tai Chi turns the body into a dam that contains the Qi, in the same way that the reservoir behind a dam is quiet and peaceful so that energy can be released to drive mighty turbines that power cities.

Daoyin exercises had always been directed internally, but if they were to be performed as a martial art, then awareness of the environment and what was going on around you became critical. In a sense the martial art element of Qigong allows us to regain something that we lost when we became 'civilised': that connection to the environment that supports our very existence.

For many centuries Tai Chi was a temple art known to only a few initiates. Obviously, from time to time it would have been taught to people outside the temples and practitioners would also have left the monastic life, taking their arts with them.

Three students of Tai Chi were to be tested on their knowledge and application of Tai Chi. Their master told them to meet him at a certain place and time in the countryside. When the students arrived they found that they were at the foot of a very narrow ravine. At the head of the ravine they could see their master, but between them and their master was a powerful wild stallion grazing on the grass. Obviously the test was to get past the stallion to the master.

The first student felt confident that he could handle the stallion, and approached it in fighting stance. As he expected, the horse attacked, but with a very skillful series of blows and parries the student was able to pass the horse and reach the master without injuring himself or the horse. On his arrival the master said nothing which indicated failure.

The second student was much more apprehensive—having seen the ferocity with which the horse attacked, he doubted his ability to handle it. Anyway, he was certainly not going to do better than the first student that way. Looking carefully, he saw that if he climbed the steep sides of the ravine there was a narrow ledge that might just be out of reach of the horse. The second student therefore used his balance and stability to climb up the ravine and slowly work himself past the horse, which reared and pawed the sides of the ravine in an attempt to dislodge him. Eventually he worked his way past to the master, but again the master said nothing.

The third student simply strolled casually into the ravine. The horse, sensing neither fear nor aggression, simply ignored him—it was he that was congratulated by the master.

At one level this story shows us three levels of martial arts. The lowest skill is to use physical skills to defend yourself. The second lowest skill is to avoid the conflict. The highest level skill is to create the conditions in which the conflict does not arise.

In case this does not sound very 'real life', consider a study done with New York prison inmates who had committed apparently random attacks on victims. They were shown pictures of people walking down alleyways and asked to nominate which ones they would attack. The results showed that while the offenders had no idea why they selected some people as victims, a pattern emerged. If the victim who walked through the alleyway looked nervous, ill at ease or displayed signs of physical weakness, this vulnerability would be sensed and an attack would ensue. If the victim displayed an aggressive or confrontational attitude this would also be sensed and again an attack would ensue. If, on the other hand, the victim simply looked at home in the environment, comfortable and relaxed, then there was no trigger and no attack. Readers are cautioned that this study is only valid for 'random' assaults—walking into a dark alley wearing a very expensive watch is not safe, no matter how relaxed and comfortable you are!

With the establishment of the foreign Ching Dynasty (1644–1912CE), temples became the centre of resistance. After some of these were destroyed, secret societies that valued new martial arts techniques, particularly those that did not require you to carry around weapons, began to develop. These secret societies were not much interested in the health aspects of the forms and not at all interested in the human development potential. They had a political agenda and focused on the pugilistic aspects. Eventually the forms became associated with prominent families such as the Chen Family and the first recognised form of Tai Chi. This was followed by the Yang Family, who eliminated the more strenuous and physically demanding techniques so that the forms could be practised by the Mandarin and educated classes.

Thus while Tai Chi had got a foothold through martial arts, the more it was practised, the more people saw that this soft, slow, flowing meditative movement technique was useful to more than martial artists. Hundreds of thousands began to try out these fascinating techniques. Here was a way of getting fit without getting hurt, a way of exercising without being bored, an art that you could benefit from in a few casual exercise sessions a week or one that you could explore to greater and greater depths for a lifetime.

Scientific studies were carried out and they found that you could practise exercises like Tai Chi and gain a level of fitness not significantly different from the most arduous and demanding of sports, without raising a sweat. Studies have also shown that Tai Chi significantly lowers the risk of falls and injury, improves the immune system, combats depression and increases the ability to focus and concentrate. Those who relax and remove stress through practising Tai Chi then take longer to become stressed again than those who relax through other means. Each new study seems to reveal a new benefit.

What has Tai Chi got against it? Well, anyone can do it and it has no 'belts' or competitive levels, so you can't do much for your ego if you want to put yourself above others. It also requires no fancy equipment, so you can't make a fortune out of manufacturing and selling it. You don't have to pay a fortune to learn mantras or acquire special knowledge. It is so flexible that it can be used for martial arts, health, as a specific therapeutic technique or for spiritual development. Tai Chi cannot be corralled for the narrow use of those who would wish you to use it the way they think it should be used— it can emerge under many new names and forms. Truly, in Tai Chi terms, the name that can be named is not the eternal name.

WEAPON FORMS

The practice of weapon forms is useful not only for martial arts applications but also for Qigong. We can explore some of these aspects by looking at sword techniques, specifically those using the Wen Jen or 'scholars' sword'. When practising this instrument one must learn to extend one's Qi through the sword as well as through the body. One must learn that the sword has a point, a sharp cutting edge close to the point, and a thick blocking edge close the hilt, and learn to direct the Qi through these various areas of the sword.

With practice one gains an appreciation of how the body and sword work together. If the mind tries to direct the sword without understanding the nature of the sword, the movements become forced and unnatural. The connection between the hand and the sword reveals itself as a new joint, a joint that must be kept open and flexible. To grip the sword too tightly is to allow your opponent to control you through the sword. The ability to listen with the sword, to sense pressure and redirect it, is a key element. The sword also reveals defects in movements and control that are too small to notice when only the hand is involved.

When practising sword techniques such as the yin-yang sword (a sword form that uses both fast and slow movements), some people are surprised at how much work is done with the sword in the left hand before the sword is moved to the right, fighting arm (this is done in reverse by left-handed people). These techniques help balance the development of the body, ensuring that the physical and energetic structure of one side does not become overemphasised. Another technique that helps ensure that the body remains balanced and harmonised is having the empty hand carried in the 'sword fingers' position: curl the little finger and ring finger towards the palm, place the pad of the first segment of the thumb across the nails of these two fingers and straighten the first and second fingers so they extend in a direct line away from the hand.

In weaponless exercise forms various breathing techniques such as 'breathing through the heels' are used to help activate energy flows while encouraging deep diaphragmatic breathing. In sword meditation, one tries to visualise energy flowing inwards through the sword on the in-breath and outwards through the sword on the out-breath.

More than anything else, the person seeking to master the sword must learn to be calm and focused. The sword is a defensive rather than offensive weapon, and the ability to wait until the opponent moves first is most important. This is often seen in Samurai sword techniques where the person who strikes first is the one who is seen as at a disadvantage. The person who has the stronger sense of centre can outwait the weaker opponent, the first strike often being initiated by the person whose focus and centre is failing them. In the yin-yang sword form this sense of centre and focus requires that the Qi is sunk and the Shen raised (see page 59).

Each weapon or instrument can teach us a little more about ourselves as we learn to work with the potential of the weapon but also within the weapon's limitations. The Broadsword, the Flying Stars, the Bamboo Pole, the Spear and many specialised weapons forms such as the Dragon Phoenix Fan, the Flute and the Ermei needles, all have a special magic all of their own.

TEN SELECT QIGONGS—A TAOIST APPROACH

Up to this point I have used a relatively systematic, analytical approach associated with western tradition to explain the nature and benefit of internal Qigong forms. In the next ten examples I use a more intuitive, Taoist approach to help you further understand the techniques of internal Qigong.

The Taoist philosophy evolved through observing nature, discerning the basic principles revealed in the external environment, and applying these principles to humankind. Often these principles were grasped intuitively rather than rationally. The following pictures are not 'illustrations' for the surrounding words; they are the 'message', and the words attached are simply aids to help you understand the picture. The principles I have selected are those I consider most important. They come from the *Tao Te Ching*, the Tai Chi Ching classics and some of the favourite sayings of my own teachers.

1. 'PRACTISE THE ART OF THE WINDBLOWN WILLOW'
The trailing limbs of the willow do not resist the wind but float upon it. Consequently, the willow tree is still standing after a storm has felled many a mightier tree.

THE HIGHEST SKILL IS HARDLY NOTICED BECAUSE IT SHOWS
NO TRACE OF EFFORT. SO IT IS WITH TAO.

Tao Te Ching

2. 'ACHIEVE STILLNESS IN MOVEMENT AND MOVEMENT IN STILLNESS'

To be still is not to be stagnant. To relax is not to collapse. To understand 'sung' and 'sinking the Qi', understand the lake. When water seeks the lowest point this is not emptiness but fullness. Neither is the water of the lake stagnant, for it is movement within stillness. The lake is like the pregnant void:

> CONSIDER THE LAKE.
> STILL ON THE SURFACE IT MOVES WITHIN.
> ITS MOVEMENT CREATES NO SOUND.
> ITS MOVEMENT HAS NO FORM.
> STILL, SOUNDLESS, FORMLESS, IT CREATES AN OCEAN OF LIFE.
> *Tao Te Ching*

3. 'RIDE THE WIND'

The Tai Chi Ching classics say, 'To ride the wind, suspend the headtop. This will be as the rising air under the eagle's wings.' Do not underestimate this power—it will support you mentally, emotionally, spiritually and physically. This is a truth discovered by meditators across the world.

> THE UNDISCERNING ARE ENTICED BY THAT WHICH IS NEW AND STRANGE.
> BUT THE SECRETS OF TAO LIE WITHIN THE ORDINARY.
> THAT WHICH IS EASILY SEEN HAS LITTLE VALUE.
> THAT WHICH HAS VALUE IS EASILY OVERLOOKED.
> *Tao Te Ching*

4. 'MOVE LIKE A GREAT RIVER'

A broad river looks like a mirror. Its power is not visible until you watch a branch whisked away on its surface or speculate on what carved the landscape that surrounds you.

THERE IS NOTHING SOFTER THAN WATER YET IT WEARS AWAY THE HARDEST ROCK.
WE SEE THIS EVERY DAY BUT FAIL TO USE THIS PRINCIPLE IN OUR OWN LIVES.

Tao Te Ching

5. 'HAVE THE STILLNESS OF A GREAT MOUNTAIN'

Nothing has the power to move and create like that which is still. Think of the great mountain ranges and how they influence the weather patterns creating their own climate and environment. Consider the cyclone, typhoon and whirlpool—each is powerful in proportion to the area of stillness at its centre. Stillness and movement are inseparable.

DAY AND NIGHT, LIGHT AND DARK, SUMMER AND WINTER.
LIFE DEPENDS ON THE INTEGRATION OF OPPOSITES.

Tao Te Ching

6. 'WALK LIKE A CAT'

The cat achieves poise and balance by separating the acts of foot placement and weight transfer. If this is important for a four-legged animal, how much more important is it for a two-legged one? We also see an effortless, gliding grace in the image of a cat.

THE HIGHEST SKILL LOOKS EASY.
LIKE TAO IT FLOWS WITHOUT EFFORT.

Tao Te Ching

7. 'HAVE THE PATIENCE OF A CAT WAITING FOR A MOUSE'

The cat is patient and waits without effort—no fuss, no tension. It does not try to tear its way through the mousehole, nor does it pace backwards and forwards—it simply waits.

A HEAVY RAIN IS FOLLOWED BY THE SUN.
A STRONG WIND GIVES WAY TO CALM.
THE MORE FORCEFUL THE ENERGY OF TAO THE SOONER IT IS EXPENDED.
DO YOU THINK THE TAO WITHIN IS ANY DIFFERENT?

Tao Te Ching

8. 'YI TAO, YEN TAO, SOE TAO'—THE WAY OF THE MIND, THE EYES AND THE HANDS

First comes the way of the mind (Yi Tao), second the way of the eyes (Yen Tao), and third the way of the hands (Soe Tao).

The first question that those new to Tai Chi often ask themselves is 'what are my hands doing?' But the more important consideration is what your mind is doing. The mind must hold the movement, its nature and its speed. The eyes, secondly, are the windows to the 'shen' (vital spirit). They reflect the spirit with which the movement is done.

Mind is followed by spirit, with the hands and body finally expressing the intention and spirit.

9. HAVE MOVEMENT ROOTED IN THE FEET, POWERED BY THE LEGS, DIRECTED BY THE WAIST AND EXPRESSED THROUGH THE HANDS

How many of us seek to strengthen the trunk and stems at the cost of the roots? To the Tao this is 'death at the centre'. This is easily understood from a physical perspective—what about the mental and emotional perspective?

BAMBOO BENDS BEFORE THE STORM,
WHILE THE PINE IS BROKEN IN TWO.
THE DIFFERENCE IS THE LIVING CENTRE.
Tao Te Ching

10. WHEN ONE PART OF THE BODY MOVES, ALL PARTS OF THE BODY MOVE

It is said that if a feather is placed on the outstretched arm of a person who has mastered Tai Chi, that person's body will move to adjust for the extra weight. The implication is that the body is a finely balanced system and the slightest change anywhere would ripple out through the whole system.

If you place a doll on its feet with its arms stretched forward it will fall on its nose. We remain standing when we make this movement because our core balancing muscles make postural adjustments to accommodate the change to our centre of gravity.

To transmit such changes, our body must contain no rigid tension, yet be taut enough to maintain its structure.

TAO IS THE SOURCE OF UNITY.
FROM UNITY COMES YIN AND YANG.
FROM YIN AND YANG COME ENERGY, ESSENCE AND STRUCTURE.
FROM THESE ALL THINGS IN OUR UNIVERSE ARE BORN.
DESTROY UNITY AND YOU DESTROY ALL THINGS.
Tao Te Ching

CHAPTER FIVE

WEI DAN

QIGONG

Wei Dan Qigong literally means
'external work with Qi'. In this book it refers to
techniques that change the Qi being taken in by the body rather
than modifying the existing Qi within it. Through practising Wei Dan
Qigong we learn that almost any aspect of the physical universe can be used to
connect us with the essence of the universe, and that the closer we come to achieving
such union, the more our lives are enriched and the more likely we are to achieve the
potential that lies within us.

Breathing, eating, drinking, writing, painting, healing, creating and experiencing art, and
working with the energies of our environment are all activities that can be performed as Qigongs, for
everything we do and touch is a reflection of Qi. The more we come to realise that the same principles work
in all these diverse areas, the more we come to understand the essential unity of the universe.

Such discussion can make the universe sound like a very serious place, but these Qigongs should be fun.
Don't work at Qigong—play at it. The one question you should ask yourself before going to sleep for the night
is, 'How many times did I laugh today?' Laugh from humour, laugh from delight, laugh from wonder.

In Qigong we learn to detect and ride the rivers, currents and waves of energy that are Qi. Should we not then
experience the same exhilaration with Qigongs that we generate when performing such activities as skiing, sailing
and gliding?

Perhaps Michelangelo, one of the greatest sculptors of all time, said it best when he stated that he did not so
much create his statues as release the form that was already locked inside. There are many roads to Wei Dan
Qigong, but the destination is the same for all—a journey to unlock the Tao within. The following thoughts
in the *Tao Te Ching* may guide us on our way:

'ON THE ROAD TO KNOWLEDGE WE SEEK TO LEARN THAT WHICH WE SHOULD KNOW.
ON THE ROAD TO WISDOM WE SEEK TO LEARN THAT WHICH WE SHOULD DISCARD.'

THE HIERARCHY OF NEEDS

Where should you start in your practice of Wei Dan Qigong? The 'hierarchy of needs' concept established by the famous psychologist Abraham Maslow provides one useful approach. This concept held that there are only a few broad categories of true human needs, and that they must be satisfied in the following order: food, shelter, companionship and self-actualisation (achievement of human potential).

Maslow recognised that life is not just about survival, just as health is more than the absence of sickness. Companionship (relationships) and self-actualisation (a person's development towards their potential) are necessary for a full and happy life.

Each of these areas of human needs has an associated Qigong form which, when applied to the activities involved in satisfying the need, enables those activities to be carried out in a way that will achieve the greatest human happiness. In this chapter I will take the liberty of transforming Maslow's hierarchy of needs into a 'Qigong hierarchy of needs'.

In Maslow's hierarchy the human need to breathe was ignored because this need is satisfied without taking conscious action. Nevertheless, breathing is our most critical need. We may live for weeks without eating food and for days without drinking, but we will live only minutes without breathing.

NEED	QIGONG	ACTIVITY/TECHNIQUE
AIR	BREATHING QIGONG	BREATHING MEDITATION, AWARENESS OF AND INFLUENCE UPON AIR QUALITY.
FOOD	NUTRITIONAL QIGONG	AWARENESS OF AND FOCUS UPON DIET, COOKING PRACTICES, FOOD PRESENTATION AND EATING TECHNIQUES.
	WATER QIGONG	DRINKING AND BATHING HABITS, AWARENESS OF WATER IN THE ENVIRONMENT.
SHELTER	ENVIRONMENTAL QIGONG	(FENG SHUI) AWARENESS AND UNDERSTANDING OF THE EFFECTS OF OUR SURROUNDINGS, INCLUDING THE HOME, GARDEN AND WORKPLACE.
COMPANIONSHIP	RELATIONSHIP QIGONG	UNDERSTANDING THE DYNAMICS OF QI WITHIN SEXUAL RELATIONSHIPS, FAMILY RELATIONSHIPS, COMMUNITY RELATIONSHIPS AND WORK RELATIONSHIPS.
SELF-ACTUALISATION	SELF-ACTUALISATION QIGONG ARTISTIC QIGONG HEALING QIGONG	CALLIGRAPHY, PAINTING, DANCE, MUSIC, SUSEKI, BONSAI, TEA DRINKING. ACUPRESSURE, ACUMASSAGE, MEDITATION.

This chapter will move through these applications of Wei Dan Qigong in the order of this Qigong hierarchy of needs. However, it is important to realise that there is no such rigid division between Qigongs in real life, for a Qigong often contains elements of other Qigongs (for instance, Nutritional Qigong also has healing, artistic and environmental aspects).

BREATHING QIGONG

THE NATURAL BREATH

Proper breathing can add so much to your health and wellbeing. This is the objective of Breathing Qigong. Through the action of breathing, the body tries to match the quantity of oxygen taken in with the changing oxygen needs of billions of cells. If too much or too little oxygen is taken in we may feel giddy and nauseous, or even pass out.

A natural breath is one in which you let the body determine how much air it needs. However, this does not mean that the various parts of the body get all the oxygen they need, for the circulatory system also has an important part to play. When the body is stressed, the circulatory system closes down the fine capillary network that takes blood out into the tissues. The cells may need more oxygen but there is no way for it to reach them.

Being in a relaxed state is therefore an important aspect of Breathing Qigong. Poor posture compresses body tissues and inhibits circulatory function, as does intense cold. To ensure that the air you breathe in gets to the places it is needed, relax, maintain good posture and keep warm. Massage can also be of help.

BREATHING RATE

The amount of oxygen your body needs per minute can be supplied with lots of shallow, fast breaths or a few deep, long breaths. However, both have very different effects on your body. Our breathing rate is linked to our stress response. The faster and shallower we breathe, the higher our level of stress and anxiety. Our heart rate also rises and falls with our breathing rate.

When we breathe slowly and deeply, our lung diaphragm (a sheet of muscle separating the thoracic and abdominal cavities) is given greater range of movement. This increases its massaging effect on the internal organs and assists their circulation and function.

Breathe deeply and you will naturally find yourself breathing more slowly—breathe more slowly and you will naturally breathe deeply. Focus on the feel of the air flowing in and out of your body and the sensations it causes. You may notice a gentle rise and fall of the shoulders, the movement of the scapulae up and down the back of the rib cage and the expansion and contraction of the stomach. Focusing on these sensations will make your breathing rate slow down and deepen.

THE LUNG DIAPHRAGM

The lung diaphragm is a 'semi-voluntary' muscle—it can be controlled by the conscious or the subconscious mind. The element of conscious control is of value in threatening or stressful situations, however it also gives the mind a chance to interfere with the function of the lung diaphragm. When we are emotionally stressed the lung diaphragm becomes tense and difficult to move. There are a number of exercise, visualisation and massage techniques that can be used to release tension within the lung diaphragm. These are covered in detail in another book I have written, *Tai Chi for Better Breathing*.

'You don't eat with your nose, so don't breathe with your mouth.' This rather inelegant Chinese saying makes its point—breathing in and out through the nose is the proper way to breathe (except during vigorous exercise and activity, when the body requires large amounts of oxygen). Breathing in through the nose ensures that the air reaching the lungs is properly filtered, adequately moistened and at the correct temperature, minimising the risk of infection and damage to the delicate lining of the lungs. Breathing out through the mouth means that the nose is unable to recover moisture from the moist out-breath. Over time the nose lining dries out and is unable to function correctly.

You may think that your nostrils look too large to filter out bacteria and viruses, but they are designed to create swirling air currents that bring the hapless invaders in contact with the sticky mucous-covered lining of the nose and trap them.

BREATHE IN WAVES

The movement of waves on a beach never comes to an abrupt halt, even though they change direction. This is also the way we should breathe, with gentle lung movements. Breathe in gradually, increasing the speed of the in-breath, then as your lungs begin to reach their comfortable limit, slow the breath and begin to breathe out. As the exhalation reaches its comfortable limit, slow the breath and begin to breathe in. This is referred to as 'wave breathing'.

Wave-breathing reduces the likelihood of over-breathing (taking in too much oxygen) and produces a smooth, gentle movement of the lung diaphragm, which is of benefit to the internal organs and will also move you towards a relaxation response.

A good training tool for this type of breathing is to visualise a straight, undisturbed candle flame positioned at a point just in front of and below your nose. Subconsciously you will be aware that any sudden changes in the airflow will cause the flame to flicker. Because the greatest change occurs at the beginning and end of your breaths, you will find that your breathing slows and softens at this point without any need for conscious direction.

THE AIR WE BREATHE

It is likely that you ensure that the water you drink is clean and fresh. Many people even buy bottled drinking water or install filters and purifiers in their household taps, but how many of us are actively concerned about the quality of the air we breathe?

Making dramatic changes—moving to live in areas alongside forests and oceans away from industrialised pollutants, for example—may not be possible, but there are things that we can do to improve the quality of the air in our homes and workplaces. An air ioniser can be used to add negative ions to the air. Plants are great detoxifiers of air, removing pollutants and carbon dioxide while preventing the air from becoming too dry. Air-purifying devices can be used to remove dust, particulates and positive ions from your air. Air circulation is also extremely important, for the quality of Qi in the air degrades if the air becomes stagnant.

BREATHE THROUGH YOUR FEET

Many people are surprised to learn that we 'breathe' through our skin as well as our lungs. The skin and lungs have the same embryologic origin. Just as oxygen and other molecules diffuse across the layers of our skin and are absorbed into the human body, so does Qi. While most of us are (sensibly) reluctant to breathe polluted air and foul-smelling odours into our bodies through our nose and mouth, we may neglect the quality of substances being absorbed into our bodies through the skin.

The ancient Chinese had an injunction that 'one should breathe through one's feet'. This means that as you breathe in and out you should visualise yourself drawing Earth Qi through your feet at the same time as you draw in Heaven Qi through your mouth, thus mixing the two. Perhaps the saying is also a recognition of the fact that our whole body breathes and that we should be mindful of all that we breathe. What, for instance are your feet breathing into your body right now?

Keep your skin clean and free of oils, waxes and any other materials that inhibit its ability to function correctly. Wear clothing that allows air circulation across the skin. Opt for wearing open sandals on your feet—if that's not practical, at least let your feet breathe free at home!

AIR QI

In chapter three we learned that the body extracts Ren (Human) Qi from a number of sources, including air. The quantity and quality of Qi in the air and our individual efficiency at extracting this Qi have a strong effect on our health, wellbeing and vitality.

Qi is of high quality and quantity when it is high in negative ions, low in pollutants and free-flowing. Aromas such as pine, peach and lemon add to the Qi of the air; putrid, chemical, or scorched/burnt aromas indicate low-quality Qi.

Located three fingerwidths below the navel is an acupoint called Qi Hai (The Sea of Qi). This point is associated with extracting Qi through the breathing process. Focus on this point by placing your hands across it or by visualising your breath reaching down to this point. This will activate the point and improve your body's efficiency in taking up Qi through the Tan Tien (see page 48).

THE INNER SECRETS OF BREATHING QIGONG

I have introduced the basic Breathing Qigong concepts of the natural breath because these alone can yield very dramatic health benefits. For those who master the 'Natural Breath' and wish to pursue the subject further, other very sophisticated Qigong breathing techniques use the abdominal muscles, the urogenital diaphragm, three spinal pumps and the application of sound, colour and other visualisations. Breathing techniques have important application to meditation and Qi circulation.

NUTRITIONAL QIGONG

Nutritional Qigong is not about eating Chinese food or using chopsticks; the concepts of nutritional Qigong can be applied to any cuisine. Nor is Nutritional Qigong about eating to maintain body shape or to cure or alleviate health conditions such as high blood pressure, diabetes, asthma and arthritis. Nutritional Qigong is about applying Qi theory to your diet to ensure that it maintains your health, happiness and longevity. It is concerned with maintaining vitality, energy, and mental, emotional and spiritual health, in addition to physical health.

Nutritional Qigong recognises that each person requires a unique diet specifically suited to them depending on their age, physical constitution, occupation, ethical and religious beliefs and the climate and season. Nutritional Qigong does not provide lists of foods and the quantities and proportions in which they should be eaten. Rather, it provides people with the knowledge and skills to ensure that their diet meets the needs of their body, mind and spirit.

This Qigong deals not only with what are the best foods are for an individual but also with the general principles of how to select, mix, cook, present and eat foods. It is comforting to realise that although the Chinese have long recognised that health is intimately related to diet, this has not prevented them from developing a cuisine based on delightful tastes, textures and appearance. Your pursuit of Nutritional Qigong should make your meals a delight to the spirit and the senses as well as the body!

THE GOLDEN AGE OF DIET

Some of the criticism of our modern diet is soundly based, but the remedy is more a matter of finetuning than harking back to a mythical 'golden age of diet' that supposedly existed sometime in prehistory. This is a dangerous myth—the average human life expectancy during these eras rarely exceeded 30 years.

Today you will find that just about any 'nutritional fact' is subject to dispute and dissension. Various experts enjoin us to eat more or less of this food group or that and threaten us with all sorts of dire consequences if we don't. You may not be aware that the health risks associated with being underweight are many times higher than those associated with being overweight.

THE POSITIVE SIDE OF DIET

Human beings thrive on an immense variety of diets in different countries and cultures. It appears to me that those countries that treat diet as an art form—something to be enjoyed and savoured rather than something to be feared—have a diet that is more successful from a health perspective. Despite the great differences between the French and Japanese diets, for example, both diets are associated with the healthiest populations in the world.

Nutritional Qigong is about developing the tastes and textures of your food, creating aroma, mixing colours and attending to presentation. The focus is not on how food may threaten your health and longevity but on how your food can make you healthy and happy in mind, body and spirit. Such an approach leads to an 'inclusive' attitude towards diet, and all aspects of acquiring, preparing and consuming your food become enjoyable in themselves. The process is unashamedly sensuous and indulgent.

Does this result in gluttony and overeating? Who are we more likely to find drunk in the gutter—the connoisseur of wine or the person who drinks without attention to a wine's colour and bouquet, without knowledge of how and where it was created, without delight in the savouring of its qualities? Nutritional Qigong seeks to turn you into a connoisseur of fine foods, a gourmet—a person whose respect and appreciation of their food is such that they could never contemplate its abuse.

A varied diet is much more likely to contain what you need. Be very careful of any diet that limits the different types of foods you are exposed to, as this is likely to limit your access to necessary proteins, minerals and vitamins.

FOOD AS FUEL

We consume food to provide the energy to power our metabolic activity. Fuelling the body is a process of balancing energy out with energy in. Too much and the extra fuel gets stored as fat. Too little and the body first begins breaking down fat and then moves on to break down muscle tissue—a process that will eventually result in death. Before the days of weighing machines we would know that we were consuming too much fuel when we started to look flabby. Now we take increases in weight as an indication that we are eating too much.

Forget average-weight-for-height-and-age tables. Finding a person with the 'correct' average weight is only slightly more likely than finding a family with the 'average' 2.6 children.

BALANCING THE CALORIE EQUATION

A calorie is a way of measuring both the energy content of food and the amount of energy an activity consumes. If we are using 3000 calories a day then we know that we need to digest at least 3000 calories a day to maintain a balance. However, without very careful monitoring it is unlikely that you could accurately estimate your daily intake to within a thousand calories. This factor alone would result in a mismatch of thirty per cent. Calorie consumption varies greatly between different body types and metabolisms, just as foods vary in their calorie content per gram— 100 grams of apple will not always equal a certain number of calories, for example.

Supposing you could accurately count the calories you are putting in your mouth, the next variable is the efficiency of your digestion, that is, how many calories you actually digest. This varies dramatically between individuals and changes as we age. Digestive efficiency depends a great deal on the health of various bacteria that colonise our guts. The percentage of calories absorbed from your food rises and falls with the health of those bacterial colonies. So forget monitoring calories unless you are hooked up to as many monitors and controls as an astronaut.

Many so-called 'weight loss' diets appear to produce dramatic results in terms of weight loss but are in fact only adjusting fluid retention levels. These dramatic adjustments in fluid levels cannot be regarded as weight loss, are not permanent and carry significant health risks.

The Nutritional Qigong approach to the fuel element of diet is simple, practical and provides a true picture of your current individual calorie equation, helping you keep the balance by making only small adjustments when necessary. Firstly, continue to enjoy your food. If you feel that you are putting on weight and becoming overweight, slowly reduce the amount of food that you consume each day until the rate of weight increase plateaus (not falls!). Take careful note of the types and quantities of food you are eating. Then, if you wish to reduce your weight, increase your physical activity above what you would normally do or reduce your diet further, but regard these as temporary adjustments and don't aim for rapid weight loss. If you are not obese and your weight loss program is causing fatigue, depression or stress, discontinue it.

FOOD FOR THE EMOTIONS AND SPIRIT

To the modern nutritionist a calorie is a calorie, and each one has the same effect on a person regardless of the source and appearance of the food from which it is obtained. Any effect of a certain food on the mind, emotions or spirit is generally seen as a disruption to the normal chemical processes within the body.

To the Chinese, the appearance, colour, aroma and presentation of food is also important as these things reflect the nature and quantity of the Qi contained within that food. Imagine the difference between a three-course meal that consists of three exquisitely presented courses and a meal with all three of those courses dumped in the one large bowl. Though it would contain the same number of calories and the same chemicals, quite a different set of emotions and spirit would be generated.

Focus on how different meals affect your emotions and spirit. Observe whether certain foods make you relaxed and calm, are uplifting, stimulating or energising. Use these foods to enhance your happiness. The yin-yang concept and the Five Elements or Five Elemental Energies theory can be applied as a Nutritional Qigong too, so it's not just a process of trial and error.

FOODS THAT GROW AND MAINTAIN THE BODY

The second reason for consuming food is to gain the materials we need to grow and maintain our bodies. In this respect modern nutritionists are primarily interested in our intake of proteins, minerals and vitamins, and the role of enzymes in building tissue and making our bodies function. Again, nutritionists are concerned with balance. The body has certain needs that must be met if it is to function correctly. However, an excessive consumption of proteins, minerals and vitamins may disrupt the metabolic function. In the same way that it is difficult to determine the number of calories each individual person needs to fuel their body, gauging the quantity of nutrients required to repair and maintain the body also proves to be problematic.

As we prepare our food we tend to assume that certain nutrients are present within it, and we often give little thought to how the nutritional content may be affected in terms of freshness. Has it been stored and transported in a fashion that maintains the nutrient value? Has it been treated with chemicals that degrade the nutrient content of the food or have negative impacts on the body and its energy systems? And we often don't think much about the changes we make to the food as we prepare it. What impact on nutritional content does the preparation or cooking process have? Do these processes degrade or enhance the nutritional content? Are the different nutrients contained within the meal compatible with each other? How does the presentation of the food, the environment where it is eaten and the physical and psychological state of the person eating and digesting the meal impact on its nutritional value?

Nutritional Qigong does not just focus on the potential nutritional value of your diet, but the actual nutritional value derived at the end of the digestive process, ensuring that you gain all the nutrients your body needs for growth and repair.

Likewise, the Nutritional Qigong approach to diet supplements is to seek out interesting, stimulating foods and include the five tastes, colours, aromas and textures in your diet. This leads to a varied diet, which is the best guarantee of avoiding deficiencies of those elements required for the proper growth and repair of the physical body.

NUTRITIONAL QIGONG AND THE YIN-YANG CONCEPT

Foods that 'heat up' or 'dry out' the body are considered yang in nature, for they increase and stimulate the flow of Qi. Foods that 'cool down' or 'moisten' the body slow and calm the flow of Qi, and are therefore considered to have a yin nature. Nutritional Qigong uses this concept to adjust the body's energy.

Without realising it, you probably already use this approach in your diet. Consider, for instance, how our diet consists of more salad and fruits in summer and more warm soups and stews in winter. In Nutritional Qigong terms, we are making our diet more yin in the summer to balance the more yang environmental conditions, and more yang in the winter to balance the more yin conditions.

Descriptions of 'cooling' or 'heating' foods do not relate to the temperature of the food at the time of ingestion but to the effect they have on the body's energy system. Thus, despite the fact that they are served hot, the teas drunk in the west have a predominantly cooling effect, and alcohol, despite the fact that it is most often served cold, has a predominantly heating effect.

If certain foods 'heat' or 'cool' the physical body, then under Qi theory it can be anticipated that they have a similar heating or cooling effect on the mind, emotions and spirit. It should therefore come as no surprise that some foods stimulate us mentally while other foods have a calming effect.

FOOD AND THE FIVE ELEMENTS CONCEPT

The application of the Five Elements concept to Nutritional Qigong allows us to finetune our knowledge of the effects of foods. Foods are associated with one of the Five Elements on the basis of taste, colour and appearance. Since foods of a particular element have stronger effects on the organs and energy systems related to that element, this technique allows us to use diet to strengthen or moderate the energy and function of particular organs.

In addition to this, specific emotions are associated with each internal organ, so the Qi from food energy will support or moderate that emotion too, and different moods will result from the consumption of different meals.

PRACTISING NUTRITIONAL QIGONG AT THE FIVE ELEMENTS LEVEL

Foods are associated with particular elements according to their taste, colour or aroma.

	TASTE	ELEMENT	ORGAN SYSTEM	FOOD EXAMPLE
GREEN	SOUR	WOOD	LIVER AND CLEANSING SYSTEMS.	LEMON, SOUR PLUM, APPLE, GRAPE, MANGO, PEACH, PINEAPPLE

SOUR FOODS SOLIDIFY THE CONTENTS OF THE DIGESTIVE TRACT.

	TASTE	ELEMENT	ORGAN SYSTEM	FOOD EXAMPLE
RED	BITTER	FIRE	HEART AND CIRCULATORY SYSTEM.	HOPS, CHIVES, GARLIC, GINGER, ONIONS, BASIL, PEPPERMINT, SOYBEANS

BITTER FOODS DRY THE SYSTEM AND PURGE THE BOWELS. BITTER IS THE MOST YIN OF FLAVOURS. IT REDUCES FEVER, CLEARS HEAT AND CALMS THE SPIRIT.

	TASTE	ELEMENT	ORGAN SYSTEM	FOOD EXAMPLE
YELLOW	SWEET	EARTH	SPLEEN AND DIGESTIVE SYSTEM.	HONEY, CHICKEN, PEANUTS, ABALONE, WHITE SUGAR, WATERMELON, SOYBEANS, MILK

SWEET FOODS DISPERSE STAGNANT ENERGY, PROMOTE CIRCULATION AND HARMONISE THE STOMACH.

	TASTE	ELEMENT	ORGAN SYSTEM	FOOD EXAMPLE
WHITE	PUNGENT/	METAL	LUNGS AND RESPIRATORY SYSTEM.	GINGER, HOPS, SPICY LETTUCE, COFFEE, ASPARAGUS, VINEGAR, WINE, GRAPEFRUIT

SPICY FOODS DISPERSE ACCUMULATED TOXINS, STIMULATE THE FLOW OF QI AND DRY MUCUS. PUNGENT/SPICY IS THE MOST YANG FLAVOUR.

	TASTE	ELEMENT	ORGAN SYSTEM	FOOD EXAMPLE
DARK BLACK/BLUE	SALTY	WATER	KIDNEY AND ELIMINATIVE SYSTEMS.	SEAWEED, CRABS, CLAMS, HAM, KELP, BARLEY, MUSSELS, KIDNEY

SALTY FOODS SOFTEN AND MOISTEN TISSUES AND FACILITATE BOWEL MOVEMENTS.

To determine whether or not any of the Five Elements are out of balance, refer to the table above. Look at the Five Organs and see if any of the physical, emotional or spiritual aspects associated with those organs are out of balance.

Where an imbalance is noticed this can be expressed as either a deficiency or excess of that element. An imbalance may be corrected by adjusting the levels of that element or bringing the levels of the other elements in balance with that element. Consuming foods associated with an element we wish to increase will correct a deficiency in that element. Decreasing the intake of foods associated with that element will correct an excess imbalance. This does not mean increasing or decreasing the amount you eat; it means changing the proportions of element related foods within that diet.

Note that in accordance with the progressive phases of the Five Elements cycle (see chapter two, page 35), increasing your intake of foods which relate to the element preceding the one we wish to adjust will also strengthen the element we wish to adjust. Similarly, increasing your intake of foods which relate to the element following the one we wish to adjust will also weaken the element we wish to adjust. For instance, increasing your intake of Water element foods will increase Wood energy, but increasing your intake of Fire element foods will decrease Wood energy.

SELECTING FOOD THAT HAS THE BEST QUALITY QI

The fruits and vegetables that contain high-quality Qi are most often those that are consumed fresh, in season and have been grown locally using organic methods. The yin-yang nature of a fruit or vegetable's Qi is likely to be more appropriate when that food is eaten fresh, in season while locally grown produce is more likely to reflect the Qi requirements of the local environment.

Organically grown fruits and vegetables are generally smaller and much more varied in appearance than plants and fruits that have had artificial fertilisers and pesticides applied to them. While gram for gram organically grown foods have more (and higher-quality) Qi than those that have been exposed to artificial foods and pesticides, you should avoid organically grown foods that show signs of being attacked by pests. The fact that such damage has occurred is usually a sign that the quality of Qi in that food was low to begin with. In addition to this, pest damage triggers many plants to produce their own natural pesticides, and this also changes the nature and quantity of Qi. For similar reasons avoid bruised, mouldy, overripe, unhealthy-looking fruits and vegetables whether they are organic or not.

Meat, poultry and seafood contain high-quality Qi when the animal has been locally reared and raised in a situation as close to its natural environment as possible, and stored with freshness in mind. Avoid animals that have been farmed on an 'intensive' basis (ie choose free-range chicken). Locally grown animal products are stored in transit for less time and are therefore likely to be fresher. Avoid any meat, poultry or seafood that shows signs of bruising, loss of colour, or excessive dryness or moisture.

MAINTAINING THE QUALITY AND QUANTITY OF QI WHILE STORING, TRANSPORTING AND PRESERVING FOODS

There is an old Chinese adage that says you should not eat a food unless that food can rot and you should not eat the food when it does rot. Minimise all physical trauma the food is subjected to. With the exception of moist foods (which should not be allowed to dehydrate), store foods in cool, dry, dark areas. Moist foods should be stored in sealed containers.

Other methods of preservation have various effects on the quantity and nature of the Qi of the food. Sun-drying, dehydration and smoking concentrate the Qi. Pickling, salting and fermenting food can change the nature of the Qi: this can be a good thing or a bad thing, depending on your individual needs and what you want the nature of the Qi to be. Pickled, salted and fermented foods are more resistant to decay and deterioration; from the Chinese viewpoint, this resistance is a reflection of stronger Qi. The food lasts longer because it has stronger Qi. Freezing seems to be a neutral process that slows down Qi loss. Chemical preservatives should not be opposed simply because they are artificial, but because they introduce a generally unknown factor in terms of how they will affect Qi. Any ingested substance has the ability to affect your body's internal Qi.

With the exception of preserved foods, the fresher the food the better. So where possible, buy small amounts of food frequently.

PREPARING YOUR MEALS

The preparation and presentation of a meal will not increase its Qi, but it will increase the quality and quantity of Qi that is assimilated into the body when it is eaten. The sight and smell of food alone can bring a rush of saliva to our mouth and set our stomach churning. When a food appeals to our senses it triggers a response in the body, preparing it for the digestive process. If the saliva and gastric juices are not present in the right quantities at the right time, the digestion of food and the absorption of Food Chi will be less efficient. From a Nutritional Qigong perspective, it is important that food is as stimulating and enjoyable as possible and that a meal is pleasing in aroma and taste, pleasing to the eyes and pleasing to the body.

To be 'pleasing to the eyes' means more than including foods of the certain colours. The meal must look appetising, healthy and be presented in a visually pleasing way. Food presentation is an important aspect of Nutritional Qigong and of maintaining the efficiency of the digestive process. If a meal 'attracts' our attention it sets up a mood in which the meal can be savoured morsel by morsel, and the more slowly we eat, the better we digest.

To understand what 'pleasing to the body' means, we must recognise that the digestive process takes place over a number of hours. It is therefore important that the body feel relaxed and comfortable after a meal. Meals that are too hot or cold, contain irritants, or are too great in quantity are not 'pleasing to the body'. If you feel bloated and distended or have heartburn and stomach cramps, the digestive process will not be effective. The body is also 'not pleased' if you have an argument in the middle of a meal, or if you hurry, worry or try to carry out some stressful activity during a meal.

Nutritional Qigong maintains that the more the senses are pleasantly stimulated, the more favourable our impressions of the meal and the more effective our absorption of Qi into the body.

PREPARING THE MEAL INGREDIENTS

The most important meal preparation method is 'cooking': the application of heat, often in combination with other techniques, to change the nature of raw food, making it easier and more pleasant to digest. Cooked food is at a temperature closer to our body temperature. The stomach is designed to carry out its digestive functions at body temperature, and many of the chemical processes of digestion are in fact impaired at lower temperatures.

The Chinese have long believed that the most beneficial thing to eat is a broth or soup served at body temperature. In the past, even Chinese medicines have been served as stews and called soups. An ancient Chinese proverb notes:

> WHEN EATING A MEAL, FIRST DRINK SOUP SO THAT IN OLD AGE
> THE BODY WILL NOT BE HARMED.

COOKING AND THE MAINTENANCE OF NUTRITIONAL VALUE

Some people hold the opinion that cooking destroys some of the nutritional value of food. There may be truth in this but traditional Chinese medicine practitioners have pointed out that the issue is not the nutritional value of the food on the plate but the nutritional value assimilated into the body, less the energy costs of such assimilation. We never absorb the full nutritional value of the food we eat, so if cooking destroys twenty per cent of the nutritional value but our digestive efficiency improves to more than offset this, then it can be said that cooking effectively enhances nutritional value. The primary concern here is not to overcook foods, particularly vegetables.

PRESENTATION OF MEAL INGREDIENTS

The physical structure and presentation of a meal also has energetic aspects. The plate on which a meal is served, the physical layout of the food, the blending of colours, tastes and aromas all represent a multi-dimensional artform that is no less valuable for its transitoriness.

SELECTING THE MEAL ENVIRONMENT

Choose a physical environment that is pleasant and stimulating without being distracting or disturbing. Pay attention to factors such as temperature, ventilation, light, sound, comfort of seating, adequacy of space and quality of air. Try to create ambience.

THE ART OF EATING

If you talk through magnificent music, give a beautiful picture only a cursory glance or rush through a delightful garden or forest you would not expect to derive much benefit from these things. This also applies to the eating or ingestion of food. As a practitioner of Nutritional Qigong you have a responsibility to make sure that you get the best quality and quantity of Qi out of your meal. This is not a burden but a delight, however, like the creation or appreciation of any art, it requires an ability to focus on and be 'mindful' of what one is doing. As a guide:

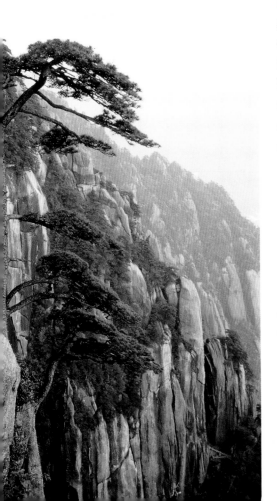

- • MAINTAIN GOOD POSTURE (RAISE THE SHEN—SEE PAGE 59).
- • BE RELAXED (SINK THE QI—SEE PAGE 59).
- • BE MINDFUL OF YOUR FOOD. FOCUS ON ITS APPEARANCE, AROMA, COLOUR, TEXTURE, MOISTNESS AND TASTE.
- • CHEW SLOWLY AND OFTEN.

After you have eaten, you can further help the digestive process by being mindful of the areas of the body where different parts of the digestive process take place. Be aware of your emotions because stress responses inhibit the production of digestion-aiding mucus. Gentle abdominal massage can be used an hour or so after a meal to aid the peristalsis action of the small and large intestines.

WATER QIGONG

THE MYSTERY OF WATER

If any substance comes close to a physical expression of our mental visualisation of Qi, it is water. We can live only days without it and even a small decrease in the levels of water within our body impacts on our energy levels and sense of wellbeing. We drink it, wash in it, breathe it, swim in it, and yet what do we really know about it? It surprises many people to find out that there are some thirty-six different 'types' of water, depending on the number and arrangement of its subatomic particles, and that these molecules form various 'structures' and patterns. We should perhaps think of water more as a liquid crystal than as a formless fluid.

Water's highly variable behaviour is physically expressed in states such as fog, snow, mist, steam and ice, in addition to its fluid nature. The Inuit people use literally dozens of names for ice to acknowledge and distinguish its different colours, textures and hardness. We need to develop the same level of discernment with respect to the water in our environment if we are to practise successful Water Qigong.

Most of us are aware that when water crystallises as a snowflake each is unique in pattern, but the creation of this pattern is not a random event. When a snowflake is melted then re-crystallised the same snowflake pattern reappears! How does the water 'remember' a complex arrangement of billions of molecules? Does water 'carry' information the

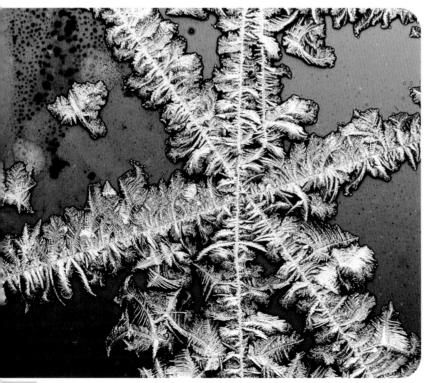

same way that radio waves carry information in the air around us? It seems that there is an energetic aspect to water that requires much further investigation. It may explain the success of healing springs and waters throughout the world, across every culture.

Considering that a large proportion of our body is composed of water (ninety-seven per cent at birth and seventy-five per cent as adults) and that water seems to carry 'information' that affects the way our body functions, it is important to ensure that the information it carries is correct—that the water we drink is of high quality.

Treat water in the same way that you treat wine. Seek out the best deep spring water and store it carefully in a cool dark place. Avoid plastic storage containers as these could leach chemicals or minerals into the water.

We need to drink about eight glasses of fresh water a day. Cool (not icy) water has more structure and benefit than warm water. Pouring and gently stirring water increases its quality. Savour its taste and texture.

THE YIN AND YANG OF WATER

Martial artists and meditators have long recognised the energising potential of being within a stream of falling water. Tiredness and lethargy are washed away in a moment. The negative ion content stimulates and refreshes. The spirit is lifted and we are often moved to break into song. We may not all have access to a mountain waterfall but the humble household shower or swimming at a surf beach can have a similar effect.

Bathing in still, warm water is quite different. Tensions dissolve and we feel quiet, tranquil and refreshed, but prepared for rest. Baths can be healing places and the addition of various minerals and salts can be used to strengthen this process.

Various other energetic effects can be achieved through saunas, hot tubs, flotation tanks and spas. Learn to use water as a Qigong that balances you externally as well as internally.

LIVING WITH WATER

For thousands of years mankind has built towns and cities along the edges of oceans and on the banks of rivers and streams. Where such natural features were missing, people enriched and re-energised their world with fountains, artificial waterfalls and ponds and pools of all shapes and sizes. This fascination with water is growing, with indoor water fountains and features becoming ever more popular. Consider your environment and how the addition of a water feature could add movement and sounds that would enliven your surroundings in both your house and your garden.

THE SOUNDS OF WATER

Think of the sound of rain as it falls on leaves, the sound of a stream as it rushes over rounded stones, the thunder of a waterfall, the pounding of waves and the lapping of a stream or lake. Our world is full of the sounds of water. Water produces 'white sound', that is, sound that absorbs other sound, such as traffic noise and other noise pollutants of the modern age. In Water Qigong we can use this to make our environment more enjoyable. These sounds can also be a subconcious reminder of the last time we heard this sound—near waves or waterfalls—and felt good. Such sounds can help us find our centre.

ENVIRONMENTAL QIGONG (FENG SHUI)

We do not have to eat, breathe or drink the Qi that surrounds us for it to have an effect on us. Simply living within a physical environment exposes us to the influence of its Qi. The Chinese refer to Environmental Qigong as Feng Shui (pronounced 'foong shway'), meaning 'wind' and 'water'. Wind symbolises the flow of Qi energy, and water symbolises the storage or accumulation of Qi.

In Feng Shui we really come to terms with both the universality of Qi and its pervasive impact upon our lives. When you start to understand how your life, your energy and your happiness can be influenced by the mountains and rivers around you, the climate, the size of your house, the nature of your garden and even your individual furnishings, then the distinction between you and the rest of the universe begins to blur and fade, and you begin to see all existence as one vast interconnected web of energy.

Thus Environmental Qigong involves much more than getting a Feng Shui expert to tell you what is right or wrong with the house you are living in or contemplating buying. Environmental Qigong is about becoming sensitive to the energetic nuances of your environment, learning to appreciate your environment and working with it. It adds a new dimension to your relationship with your environment and a new opportunity to balance your Qi.

In many ways, the practice of Environmental Qigong leads us to the point where we realise that the concept of an individual having energy that is influenced by the energy of the environment is in fact largely an illusion; we are really nothing more, or less, than environmental energy. To understand this, picture a river with small eddies and whirlpools. The whirlpools seem to have a separate existence, but in reality they are only artifacts created by the flow of water within the river.

The vortex whirls water molecules around for a few moments before releasing them back to the river. In the same way, we circulate the Qi (and the very atoms) that we extract from eating, breathing and drinking before releasing them back to the environment. Where the vortex itself goes depends not on the water molecules that form it but on the direction of the water within the river. In the same way, we may be more influenced by the tides of Qi in our external environment than the Qi within us.

THE ORIGINS OF FENG SHUI

The belief that stimulated the development of Feng Shui was, somewhat paradoxically for a science dealing with life energy, a concern about the siting of ancestral graves. The Chinese believed that the spirits of their ancestors played a vital and important role in the lives of their descendants. The 'stronger' the spirit, the more chance it would have to influence the descendants' lives. The best thing that the descendants could do to enhance the 'strength' of their ancestors' spirits was to ensure that their graves were well sited in relation to the flow of Qi. The development of techniques to do this became known as Yin Feng Shui. Techniques to enhance the energy of the living are now known as Yang Feng Shui.

Yin Feng Shui even became involved in military campaigns where sorties to destroy the graves of the opposing leader's ancestors (thus weakening the ancestors' powers) became common practice. Re-siting one's own ancestors' graves into a more propitious location also became part of military strategy.

Steep, rocky, angular peaks are all evidence of yang energy within the environment. Yang energy is very much associated with spiritual development. Interestingly, religions originating outside China also use yang energy in buildings such as spires, minarets, pyramids and steeples. The Taoists (being nature-based) sought out natural sources of energy to assist their spiritual development. Where such energies were not naturally available, or needed to be enhanced, they constructed pagodas and soaring roofs.

A number of approaches to the practice of Feng Shui developed over time, including:

- • - THE 'FORM' APPROACH, WHICH ASSESSED THE INFLUENCE OF QI BY LOOKING AT THE PHYSICAL CHARACTERISTICS OF THE SURROUNDINGS, INCLUDING MOUNTAINS, VALLEYS, RIVERS AND PLAINS, THE SHAPE AND CONSTITUTION OF BUILDINGS AND THEIR CONTENTS.

- • - 'COMPASS' SCHOOLS, WHICH ASSESSED THE INFLUENCE OF QI BY LOOKING AT THE NUMERICAL PROPORTIONS OF NATURE AND THE USE OF WHAT IS KNOWN AS THE FENG SHUI COMPASS OR LOPAN.

- • - ASTROLOGICAL SCHOOLS, WHICH ASSESSED THE INFLUENCE OF QI THROUGH THE DATE OF BIRTH OF INDIVIDUALS OR THE DATE OF CONSTRUCTION OF BUILDINGS, AND FOLLOWED THE UNIVERSAL CYCLES OF ENERGY AS A GUIDE TO THEIR PARTICULAR INFLUENCE AT ANY ONE POINT IN TIME.

When the Chinese communist government came to power it was opposed to such 'traditional' beliefs and tried to suppress the study of Feng Shui, particularly during the time of the Cultural Revolution. However, persecution of those practicing the skills only served to encourage the spread of Feng Shui throughout the world (see page 66).

Many of the current schools blend the techniques and approaches discussed above, and some have even absorbed some more western approaches, such as the use of dowsing. There has also been a tendency to incorporate scientific knowledge relating to the influences of light frequencies, electro-magnetic radiation, sound vibration and colour theory on human beings.

HOW FENG SHUI WORKS

Feng Shui is not magic, or a religion—it is a Qigong.

The premises upon which the form are based are simple and few in number:

- THE QUANTITY AND QUALITY OF QI IN ANY ONE LOCATION DEPENDS ON THE PHYSICAL AND ENERGETIC CHARACTERISTICS OF THAT LOCATION, THEREFORE THE QUANTITY AND QUALITY OF QI VARIES FROM LOCATION TO LOCATION.

- THE QUALITY AND QUANTITY OF QI AT A LOCATION CAN BE CHANGED BY ALTERING THE PHYSICAL AND ENERGETIC CHARACTERISTICS OF THAT LOCATION.

- THE QUALITY AND QUANTITY OF QI AT A LOCATION INFLUENCES THE QI OF LIVING THINGS WITHIN THAT ENVIRONMENT IN ACCORDANCE WITH THE PRINCIPLES OF YIN AND YANG AND THE FIVE ELEMENTS.

- THE INFLUENCE THAT A LOCATION HAS ON THE QI OF THOSE LIVING THINGS IS PROPORTIONATE TO THE TIME THAT THE LIVING THINGS SPEND IN THE LOCATION. THIS INFLUENCE ALSO VARIES IN ACCORDANCE WITH THE INVERSE SQUARE LAW WHICH STATES THAT WITH REGARD TO ELECTRICAL AND MAGNETIC FIELDS, THE ELECTRIC FIELD OF A CONCENTRATED CHARGE DEPENDS ON THE RECIPROCAL OF THE SQUARE OF THE DISTANCE FROM THE CHARGE. THE INVERSE SQUARE LAW CAN ALSO BE USED TO CALCULATE GRAVITY FIELD EFFECTS. FOR THE PURPOSES OF FENG SHUI, THIS MEANS THAT THE QI EFFECT OF ONE OBJECT ON ANOTHER DECREASES IN DIRECT PROPORTION TO THE SQUARE OF THE DISTANCE BETWEEN THE TWO OBJECTS.

The first premise is simply a restatement of the Qi theory that matter and energy conditions such light, sound and temperature are simply reflections of underlying Qi. Different locations possess different physical forms and objects that vary in size, shape, colour and weight, and different levels of heat, light, sound and movement. This simply reflects variations in the underlying Qi.

The second premise derives from the first. If you change the physical and energetic characteristics, then the underlying Qi must change too. You cannot have two differently shaped whirlpools created by identical flows of water.

The third premise simply recognises the universal nature of Qi. That is, Qi always follows the principles of yin and yang and the Five Elements. In terms of the 'fields' and 'currents' of Qi, placing a living thing inside a certain gravitational or electromagnetic field influences that living thing, as does placing it in different currents of air and water.

The fourth premise is implicit in the actions of Feng Shui practitioners, who focus on the home and the workplace, where a person spends most of their time. They assume that the closer an object is, the greater its effect on that person. Thus, a small pool in one's garden may have more Qi influence than a lake situated 20 kilometres away.

'Form-based Feng Shui' is carried out on the strength of these four premises. The 'compass' and astrological schools add other assumptions which must be taken 'on faith'; this does not mean they are wrong, but that the concepts are more nebulous and lie outside the scope of this book.

The whole point of a Qigong is that you must practise it. This is why I prefer the term 'Environmental Qigong' to 'Feng Shui', for Feng Shui is often thought to involve seeking out expert advice. There is nothing wrong with getting expert advice on Feng Shui, just as there is nothing wrong with getting expert medical advice from a doctor! However, if your health program were to consist solely of seeing a doctor when you have a problem or for an annual check-up, while you ignore factors such as diet, exercise and lifestyle, you would miss out on the benefits of positive health. Similarly, if you only take notice of Feng Shui when you develop a problem or buy a new house, you will miss out on many potential benefits and the delightful experience of becoming more in tune with your environment.

Many people are apprehensive about practising Feng Shui because so many reference books make it sound so difficult and confusing. This is because they start Feng Shui at the wrong end, trying to find problems to fix rather than looking for areas of improvement. For example:

You read in one book that having a tree in front of your front door blocks the Qi so you dig it out, only to find that you now look straight onto a road intersection. Your Feng Shui book says a good way of stopping the Sha Qi associated with a road intersection is to put a tree between your front door and the intersection, so you plant a sapling in the place where the tree was. Then you read that the tree needs to be big to block out the Sha Qi, so you remove the sapling and replace it with a well-developed, fast-growing tree. Within a few years it is towering above the house, and you read in your Feng Shui book that this is not a good thing, so you prune it extensively. Unfortunately, the tree does not take well to this and looks sickly, which your Feng Shui book tells you is bad Qi. You have the tree removed, which leaves a stump on which you place a pot containing a medium-sized tree. However, your Feng Shui book says that tree stumps are bad Qi, and you notice that your new tree has sharp, prickly leaves, which are also bad Qi. After further investigation you find that the original tree was the best Feng Shui solution!

All these difficulties arose because the focus of attention was on the problems trees can cause rather than the real issue of how to obtain the best possible quantity and quality of Qi through the front door. Focus on problems and that is what you will get. If you turn the focus around and look for areas of your life where you can improve your happiness, Feng Shui will reveal things that you can do to assist those areas. To practise Feng Shui in this manner you need to know the areas where you want improvements in your life, the changes in your Qi that need to be made to get these desired improvements, and which changes in your environment will push your Qi in the right direction.

FINDING THE OPPORTUNITY AREAS IN YOUR LIFE

The first step in ensuring that the environmental changes we make are going to improve rather than simply change our lives, is to understand the nature of the improvements we wish to make. Fortunately, the Chinese have a particularly effective tool for tracking down the issues that are preventing us from living a happy and harmonious life—the Ba Kua, which gives us eight areas in life to consider and assess.

For the Chinese, the 'eight directions' represented by the Ba Kua are not only compass directions, but energetic directions. Our lives also have eight energetic directions that can be mapped against the Ba Kua. Even if you do not practise Environmental Qigong, assessing your life using the Ba Kua may be one of the most important things you do.

Look at each area and decide whether any change is desirable. Then write down any changes you wish to make in their order of importance. The second function of the Ba Kua is to identify the areas of your home, workplace or garden where making changes will be most effective. We will look at the nature of the changes which will create the effects we want later on page 123. (Looking at your environment through Feng Shui eyes).

The important thing to remember is that each of these areas is important throughout your life. Each area must be kept in balance with the others or an imbalance (and thus unhappiness) will result. For example, if you put too much of your life energy into generating wealth, you may find that there is not enough life energy to sustain your relationships, and so on. It becomes easier to understand the Ba Kua when you look behind the meaning of the 'labels' attached to each of these life areas.

MISSION/PURPOSE

This is described as 'Career' in most Feng Shui books. I find this modern term too limiting. The ancient Chinese did not have careers—they had a function, mission or purpose in life, and I have yet to find a person today who does not maintain that their happiness would be increased by having a point or purpose.

We all have a 'purpose', but we may not be balancing the energy of our lives in a way that supports it.

KNOWLEDGE/WISDOM

This area deals with our growth and development. It is more than the simple acquisition of facts, skills and abilities—it is our growth as a human being. Consider the last ten years of your life—can you say you have grown and developed as a human being? If the answer is no, would you be happier if you felt growth had occurred? Again, the issue here is balance, and those who have acquired vast new knowledge and skills over this time at the expense of their health, family and relationships will rarely have a true sense of personal growth and an overall increase in happiness.

HEALTH

This area is concerned with our physical, mental and emotional health. The benefits are obvious—few people who are unhealthy in these respects would argue that a return to health would not make them happier. Effort must be made to exercise and eat correctly if we are to maintain a 'healthy' approach to life. The Chinese often associate this area with 'Family', because they consider it impossible to be healthy if your family is unhealthy. After all, family largely determines your diet and exercise opportunities and your exposure to stress and conflict, or alternatively, love and support. If you wish to address your health, begin by looking at the health of your family.

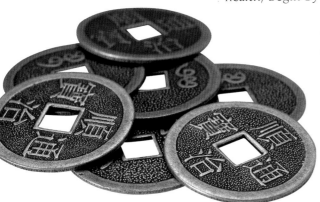

WEALTH

This is one of the most misunderstood areas. If you are living in poverty and are unable to eat properly or provide for your children, of course your happiness could be improved by more wealth, but the pursuit of wealth for its own ends unbalances our life energy. Ask yourself whether you have the wealth to live the life that you want to live. If you do you are rich, but if you do not you are poor—thus, there are many poor billionaires and many rich backpackers. The key is to know the life that will make you happiest.

REPUTATION

It used to be that a person's most valuable possession was their reputation. This concept has been largely devalued today, and replaced by 'fame', a term that conjures up the mindless adulation sought out by various celebrities. Here we are more concerned about your reputation among your spouse, your children, your relatives, your workmates and associates. Again, however, it is a matter of balance—if your reputation exceeds your abilities and you are continually being asked to do things that are beyond your capabilities and resources, this is not likely to lead to happiness either.

RELATIONSHIPS

Relationships occur in many forms. Human beings rarely need persuasion that relationships are important. Studies have shown that married couples live five years longer on average than those who do not marry. Given that many marital relationships are hardly satisfactory and that many unmarried people have strong relationships, I can't help wondering how great the difference in average life spans would be if we had statistics available on the life spans of persons with long-term positive relationships and those with no such relationships!

If we let a relationship consume too much of our life's energy, however, our other life energy areas will suffer. Again, it is a matter of balance.

CREATIVITY

This area is often called 'Children' in many Feng Shui books, but not everyone has children and those that do usually find their involvement in raising them diminishes at some point. This life area is really about our lifelong need to 'put ourselves' into something that goes beyond ourselves. While children are one such challenge, painting, music, sculpture, a business, a charity or a church can also fulfil this aspect. In essence you must 'care' for something that you use your energy to create.

ENVIRONMENT

This area is often given the rather strange label, 'Helpful people/travel'. What it really refers to is our useful connections to the environment. This aspect becomes evident when something goes wrong in life—we lose our job, have a financial crisis or a major health problem, for example. It seems that some people always have to bear up on their own while others are miraculously offered jobs, financial support or even just useful advice. The energy in this area of life is one of 'networking' with the environment. Travel plays a part in this area because it not only 'broadens the mind', but also extends our environmental contacts.

A NINTH DIRECTION?

We can move outwards from the centre in eight directions, but we can also move inwards towards the centre. This movement is considered 'the ninth direction' and refers to health—not physical health, but the health of each of the eight directions.

After we have assessed the areas of the Ba Kua, we need to express this assessment in a form that helps us understand what needs to be done. We return to the concept of yin and yang, which tells us that those areas which are too yin must be made more yang, and those areas which are too yang must be made more yin. If we can examine our environment and adjust the elements to change the energetic influence of the environment so that it supports the direction in which we want to move, we are on our way to practising Environmental Qigong.

So before making changes to the energy in any area we first need to determine whether we need to make that energy more yin or more yang. Yin life problems are reflected by a slowness and deficiency of energy—things are running down or simply not happening. Yang life problems are the reverse—too much is happening and there may be lots of conflict situations. With regards to relationships, a ying condition is indicated if you have few friendships and those that you do have are dull or tend to drift apart. If the energy is too yang in this area your relationships are more likely to explode through conflict, are exhausting or over-demanding. With regard to career, yin situations are reflected by a lack of promotion—your job seems to go on and on with no change. Long periods of unemployment could also be found. In a yang situation there is endless work to do and never enough time to do it, your work environment may seem to be one of continual change and crises.

LOOKING AT YOUR ENVIRONMENT THROUGH FENG SHUI EYES

Since our environment is very complex we need a structured way to look at the Feng Shui effects of our environment. I have developed the Eight Energy Conditions Approach to do this.

The Eight Energy Conditions are the:

- LIGHT ENERGY CONDITION
- SOUND ENERGY CONDITION
- THERMAL ENERGY CONDITION
- MOISTURE ENERGY CONDITION
- BIO-ENERGY CONDITION
- AROMA ENERGY CONDITION
- MOVING ENERGY CONDITION
- CRYSTALLISED ENERGY CONDITION.

These conditions can be studied at very sophisticated levels, but in this chapter I will only include enough to capture the essence of the energy condition and how it might be adjusted. (*Feng Shui for Personal Harmony* offers a more-detailed analysis if you wish to pursue the subject further.) It is important to remember that all these 'conditions' are really telling us about the 'condition' of the underlying Qi. When we create new 'conditions' we will have changed the underlying Qi, and the effects that this underlying Qi has on our personal Qi.

THE LIGHT ENERGY CONDITION

The Light Energy condition refers to the quantity and quality of electromagnetic energy in the environment. As such, it covers the frequency and intensity of invisible light, and the full electromagnetic spectrum, including infra-red, ultraviolet, radiowaves and microwaves. Graphic art used within the environment may also contribute to the Light Energy condition.

With respect to this condition you can make your environment more yin by:

- DECREASING THE NUMBER OR SIZE OF WINDOWS AND OTHER LIGHT SOURCES, OR USING SHADES, DRAPES OR BLINDS.
- REDUCING THE AMOUNT OF LIGHT ENTERING THE PREMISES BY TINTING, FROSTING OR STAINING GLASS WINDOWS.
- INCREASING THE USE OF LIGHT-ABSORBENT FURNITURE AND FITTINGS.
- INCREASING THE USE OF SUBDUED COLOURS.
- PLANTING SHADE TREES OUTSIDE AND ERECTING SHADE SCREENS TO REDUCE THE AMOUNT OF LIGHT ENTERING THE ENVIRONMENT.
- DECREASING THE NUMBER AND SIZE OF MIRRORS AND CRYSTALS IN THE ENVIRONMENT.
- ENSURE ARTWORK IN THE ENVIRONMENT DEPICTS PASSIVE OR TRANQUIL SCENES, IS NOT TOO BRIGHT, HAS REDUCED COLOUR CONTRAST, LESS ANGULAR STRUCTURE AND USES CURVED LINES.

You can make your environment more yang by reversing all of the above.

The quality of Light Qi can be changed in a number of ways. Crystals can change negative (Sha) Qi to positive (Sheng) Qi by dispersing overly strong flows of light. The leaves of trees and plants or their reflections on water surfaces can have similar effects. The frequencies of light that are most beneficial to human health are those contained in natural sunlight. Many artificial sources of light, particularly fluorescent lights, lack the light frequencies (spectra) found in sunlight. In essence, they are missing necessary Qi. Full spectrum lights which contain all the frequencies of natural sunlight are now available and from a Feng Shui point of view, are much more beneficial than fluorescent sources.

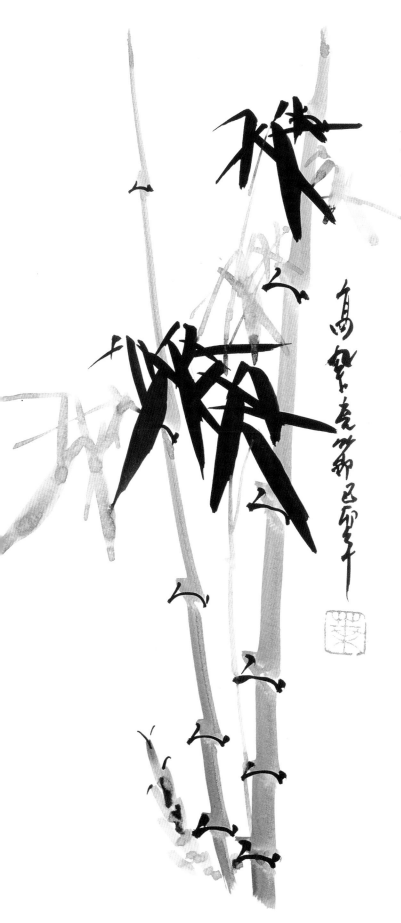

THE SOUND ENERGY CONDITION

This energy area includes all the pressure waves that travel through our physical environment, whether they be subsonic, audible or ultrasonic. The presence and use of music is also an important consideration.

With respect to this condition you can make your environment more yin by:

- INCREASING THE AMOUNT OF INSULATION OR SOUND-ABSORBING MATERIAL.
- PLACING 'WHITE SOUND' SOURCES BETWEEN YOU AND A SOURCE OF DISRUPTIVE NOISE.
- INCORPORATING SOME FORM OF A FOUNTAIN AND/OR WATERFALL.

You can make your environment more yang by reversing all of the above.

The quality of Sound Qi can be changed through the use of wind chimes, setting up an environment that attracts birds and pleasant-sounding insects such as bees, adding water sounds by incorporating fountains and artificial waterfalls, growing plants that 'capture' the sound of wind and rain near windows, and playing appropriate music. When using music to change the quality as opposed to quantity of sound, the sound must be appropriate to the change that you want to make. That is, if you want to make your condition more yang, use high-pitched, lively music with a fast beat; if we want to make your condition more yin, use music with the opposite characteristics.

THE THERMAL ENERGY CONDITION

We are natural Feng Shui practitioners in this regard. We choose to wear warm clothing and use heating in our homes and workplaces when the weather is cold, and wear light clothing and use a fan or air-conditioner when it is warm. Making changes to thermal conductivity can also change the nature of the Qi effect of the environment. Thermal conductivity relates to the speed at which heat moves through an object. For instance, if you put a cloth and a tin can in the freezer for an hour, both will be the same temperature but the can will feel colder when you touch it because it will take up the heat from your skin much faster. In the same way, stepping onto a carpet rather than a stone floor feels 'warmer', even though the temperature may be the same.

With respect to this condition you can make your environment more yin by:

- Increasing shade.
- Increasing thermal insulation.
- Increasing use of cool colours.
- Adding fountains and pools.
- Using building materials that have low thermal conductivity, such as rock and stone.
- Decreasing air circulation and flow if the outside environment is warmer or, alternatively, focusing on circulating internal air.
- Increasing air circulation where the outside environment is cooler.

You can make your environment more yang by reversing all of the above. The quality of Thermal Qi can be changed by choosing natural heat sources in the form of sunlight and insulation rather than heat from combustion and electrical devices.

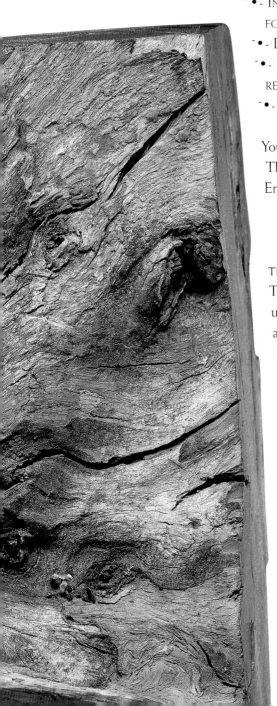

THE MOISTURE ENERGY CONDITION

The moisture level in an environment is an important indication of the state of the underlying Qi. With respect to this condition you can make your environment more yin by:

- INCREASING THE AMOUNT OF VEGETATION, PARTICULARLY TREES WITH DENSE FOLIAGE COVER.
- DECREASING AIR-FLOW.
- INCREASING EXPOSED WATER SURFACES THROUGH USE OF AQUARIUMS, REFLECTION POOLS, INTERNAL WATERFALLS AND FOUNTAINS.
- INCREASING USE OF WATER-ABSORBING MATERIALS SUCH AS WOOD AND TIMBER.

You can make your environment more yang by reversing all of the above.
The quality of Moisture Qi can be affected by the quality of water in the vicinity. Ensure that all water elements are fresh and never stagnant.

THE BIO-ENERGY CONDITION

The living things in your environment are a very strong representation of the underlying Qi. While the energetic influence can be powerful, look at the nature and physical and emotional health of the plants, animals and people that you bring into your environment.

With respect to this condition you can make your environment more yin by:

- DECREASING THE NUMBER OF LIVING THINGS WITHIN IT.
- SHIFTING THE BALANCE FROM ACTIVE LIFE FORMS TO LESS ACTIVE LIFE FORMS (FOR EXAMPLE, FISH AND PLANTS INSTEAD OF MAMMALS AND BIRDS).
- SURROUNDING YOURSELF WITH CALM, RELAXED, TRANQUIL PEOPLE.

You can make your environment more yang by reversing all of the above.
The quality of Bio-energy Qi can be changed by ensuring the health and vitality of the plants and animals in your environment.

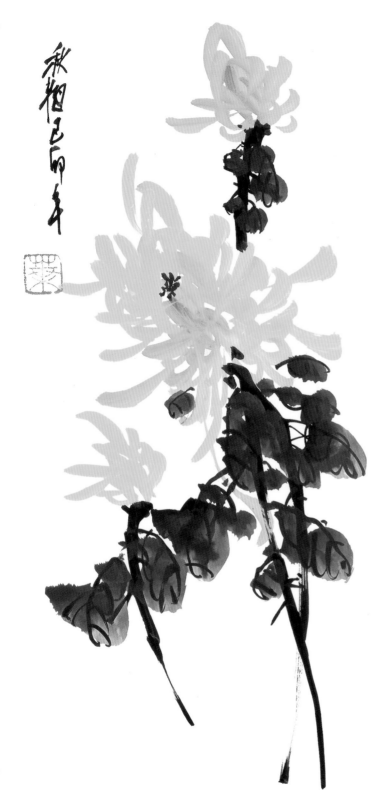

THE AROMA ENERGY CONDITION

The smells and aromas within your environment can be very powerful indicators of the underlying Qi. The most powerful aroma effect comes from the aromas that we place close to us, such as scents and perfumes.

With respect to this condition you can make your environment more yin by:

- INCREASING THE USE OF AROMAS THAT CREATE A RELAXED, TRANQUIL FEELING.
- DECREASING THE USE OF AROMAS THAT STIMULATE AND ENERGISE.

You can make your environment more yang by reversing all of the above.

The quality of Aroma Qi can be changed by eliminating bad aromas at their source rather than masking them with another aroma, and by sourcing aromas from natural rather than artificial chemical sources.

THE MOVING ENERGY CONDITION

The amount of movement occurring in our environment is a good indicator of the underlying Qi. This includes the movement of vehicles, people, plants and animals, but also that of air and water.

With respect to this condition you can make your environment more yin by:

- CREATING WINDBREAKS USING VEGETATION, FENCES OR WALLS.
- REDUCING THE USE OF STRAIGHT, NARROW PASSAGEWAYS AND PATHWAYS.
- REDUCING THE USE OF IMAGES AND ARTIFACTS THAT DENOTE POWERFUL, FAST MOVEMENT.
- INCREASING THE USE OF HEAVY, SOLID FURNITURE.
- REDUCING THE USE OF MOVING ITEMS SUCH AS FANS, WIND CHIMES, FOUNTAINS, WATERFALLS, MOBILES AND PENDULUM CLOCKS.

You can make your environment more yang by reversing all of the above.

The quality of Movement Qi can be changed by creating gentle, repetitive movement rather than jerky, irregular movement, and by sourcing movement from natural rather than artificial sources.

THE CRYSTALLISED ENERGY CONDITION

This refers to the expression of Qi as physical objects and landforms within our environment.

With respect to this condition you can make your environment more yin by:

- PHYSICAL STRUCTURES AND FURNITURE BEING SOFT, ROUNDED, MASSIVE IN FORM AND DARK IN COLOUR.
- MAKING ROOMS AND AREAS SMALLER.

You can make your environment more yang by reversing all of the above.

The quality of Crystallised Energy Qi can be changed by reducing clutter, keeping objects in tidy, well-organised arrangements and making sure that all objects are in good repair and well maintained.

CREATING AN ENVIRONMENTAL CHANGE PLAN

These examples are only some of the hundreds of changes that can be made in respect to each energy condition. Do not make too many changes at once. Decide on one or two changes to begin with and note the effect that these have on your life.

Be careful not to make any extreme changes that would create a Sha Chi or Si Chi condition. For example, if you decide to make your environment more yin by reducing the light level, don't reduce it so much that it strains your eyesight and you fall over objects. Commonsense and your own intuition are very good indicators of the degree of change required.

What do you do if different people living in the one location have different 'personal energy objectives'? The answer lies in another use of the Ba Kua, which enables you to determine which areas of your house or workplace will have the strongest influence on particular individuals and particular life areas. This is not within the scope of this book, but is explained in detail in another book I have written, *Feng Shui for Personal Harmony*.

ADVANCING YOUR KNOWLEDGE OF ENVIRONMENTAL FENG SHUI

What has been introduced in this book is the basic methodology of Feng Shui or Environmental Qigong. You should now understand how to approach this Qigong and how this Qigong relates to other Qigongs. There are many additional techniques and considerations that one can add to the basic approach outlined, including:

- How the shape and internal layout of your house can influence your Qi.
- How to determine the Qi of your local rather than immediate environment, and the implications of this for the Qi of your immediate environment.
- How the influence of the various landforms and symbolic re-creations of such landforms in your garden can influence your Qi.
- How the energetic considerations relating to colours and frequencies of light can affect you.
- The universal cycles of Qi and how your birthdate is a guide to the nature of Qi that will support you.

Do not be daunted by the fact that you are at the beginning of the road rather than the end, for the important thing is that you are 'on the road'. Like any other Qigong, take Feng Shui or Environmental Qigong step by step.

THE QI OF LANDFORM
Our personal energy (Ren Qi) is influenced by how we are located in relation to the waves of form in our environment. The energetic influence of areas at the top of mountains is very different from that found in valleys, as is the influence of the open plains and those areas in the shelter of the mountainsides. All landscapes are a reflection of the underlying Qi, whether they are naturally or artificially created.

WIND AND WATER
The physical substance of the landscape is but one aspect of the energy of the environment. Physical substance is carved and moulded by wind, water and temperature, and our location in relation to these energy flows 'carves' our Ren Qi much more easily than it carves the landscape in which we live.

CLIMATE
Climate is the result of the interaction between landscape, winds, waters and temperature. It is the result of colliding energies, and as such is energy itself. When selecting a location, the natural climate of the area should be given strong consideration.

THE QI OF HOME

THE LIVING HOME

View your house as a living organism that feeds on the energy that surrounds it and disposes of its waste products. Thus, a house must access energy through doors and windows or have energy-generating sources such as heating and lighting devices brought within. The energy of a house should flow plentifully and not be stagnant.

THE SENSUAL HOME

Our senses detect the energy of light, the energy of sound, the energy of aroma and the energy of form. All these energies interact with—and transform—our personal energy. As in all things, we must seek balance and create a home that energises but does not exhaust us. Because different areas of a house are used for different activities, each area requires different energies for support.

THE ENERGETIC HOME

Consider the nature of the energy you bring into your home. The artificial light you generate, your own emotional state when you enter the house, the music you play and the nature of the images placed on the walls as pictures or introduced through television and computer screens all represent energy patterns and have different levels of influence.

THE BA KUA HOME

The form and structure of your home affects its internal energy structure. This means that the energy of some areas of the house will be more suited to supporting the energy of some activities. These energies can be determined using the Ba Kua. The many different house designs and layouts mean that any of the rooms discussed below may fall within any of the Ba Kua life areas. The Qi of a room must support its function first and then the Ba Kua life area. For instance, if your bedroom is located within the Wealth area, it would be counterproductive to increase the energy in the Wealth area to the degree that it disturbs your sleep patterns. This could well result in poor health, loss of concentration and poor decision-making—none of which is very likely to improve your wealth!

THE QI OF BEDROOMS

The energy of a bedroom needs to support sleep. The energy should be calming and non-disturbing. Of course relationship energy must also be considered and this has contrasting energy requirements. The use of light, colour and aroma can be used to create different energies at different times and different energies within different places in the room. Thus we can find ways of supporting the different energies of two people even if they are sleeping in the same bed.

THE QI OF DINING ROOMS

We often rush our meals or substitute them with a simple snack eaten on the run. Even monks, who give up many of life's pleasures, retain the practice of dining. An eating area should be free of distraction, allowing people to focus on the meal. The setting should be one that creates a feeling of calmness and serenity.

Mealtimes can also be used to strengthen family relationships. Enhancing energies that encourage communication (such as having a round rather than square table and using orange colours) can help achieve this.

THE QI OF LIVING ROOMS

The living room should create energy that supports the family's activities and games. Families have quiet times and active times, so the energy of the room needs to be variable. There will also be different age groups and different interests whose energies need to be catered for. Entertaining also requires a different level of energy. Perhaps because of this, we tend to see 'family' rooms in houses these days as well as more formal entertaining areas.

THE QI OF KITCHENS

The Qi of the kitchen must promote the vitality of the Qi of all food stored and prepared in the area. It is also important that the energy of the kitchen supports the preparer of food. Be aware of the negative energy that clutter can bring. Kitchens contain Sha Qi in the form of sharp knife blades and very hot areas. Managing the energy of a kitchen is a challenging task, but efforts made here are well rewarded.

THE QI OF BATHROOMS AND LAUNDRIES

Bathrooms are unnecessarily maligned in many Feng Shui books. The bathroom is as necessary to a house as our kidneys and eliminative organs are to our bodies. The energy of this area is not bad, it simply requires scrupulous attention to ensure that it remains healthy. Thus bathrooms and laundries should be kept light, dry, warm, colourful, well aired and free of clutter.

THE QI OF OFFICES AND STUDIES

An office or study should suit the energetic requirements of the activity. If the room is used for the purposes of study and accumulating knowledge, then the study should be yin in nature—quiet and non-distracting. If the area is a home office, however, the study should be more colourful and stimulating, with a yang nature to foster creativity and action.

THE QI OF GARAGES

Garages are notorious areas for accumulation of clutter, which causes energy stagnation. Motor vehicles also continue to produce volatile chemicals while they cool down. Every effort should be made to keep the garage clutter free and well ventilated, but it is probably best if the energy of this area is isolated from the rest of the house. Rooms above a garage should have an impermeable floor. If a garage door connects to the house it should be self-closing and open inwards to the garage.

THE QI OF GARDENS

MOUNTAINS IN YOUR GARDEN

You may live hundreds of kilometres away from mountains but you can still bring mountain energy into your garden through the use of rocks and the creation of artificial mountains such as rockeries. These anchor Qi to your land.

RIVERS IN YOUR GARDEN

Again, you may live far away from the nearest river or lake but you can create the energy of moving water in your garden by adding a stream, pond or artificial fountain. Such features add energy to your garden and generate white 'sound', which absorbs and masks Sha Qi sound. Water invites life into your garden in the form of aquatic life, birds, frogs and insects. (Noxious insects are usually only a problem if the water is allowed to stagnate.)

THE FIVE ELEMENTAL ENERGIES IN YOUR GARDEN

The garden is a good place to balance the Five Elemental energy phases. This can be done through the use of symbols, colours, and shapes related to the Five Elements.

The table below can be used as a guide to show which factors relate to which element. To obtain the correct 'positions' listed in the table, take all directions from the vantage point of standing at the centre of your property facing towards the front entrance.

POSITION	ELEMENT	SYMBOL	COLOUR	SHAPE
left	Wood	dragon	green	columnar
front	Fire	bird	red	pyramidal
centre	Earth	snake	yellow	cubical
right	Metal	tiger	white	spherical
rear	Water	turtle	black	irregular

THE QI OF PATHWAYS

Pathways redistribute the energy of your garden and can be used to highlight various aspects and features. The straighter, wider and smoother the pathway, the greater and faster the flow of Qi along it. Incorporating curves (particularly around water features) will slow down the flow of Qi. Therefore, if you have a Ba Kua area of your land that requires more Qi movement, consider adding a pathway or making the existing pathway straighter, wider and smoother. If you want to reduce the movement of energy, remove the path or make it more smooth, narrow and windy.

THE QI OF PLANTS AND FLOWERS

The Qi of a plant or flower is expressed through its colour, aroma, and the shape and texture of its leaves and stems. Observe closely and you will see that different foliage creates wave motions of quite different natures. Thus the Chinese differentiate between such things as 'willow waves' and 'pine waves'. Leaves that move and rustle in the slightest breeze are said to 'invite' the wind, and enhance the feeling of movement within a garden. Similarly, certain leaves 'invite' the rain—the sound of rain falling on the leaves of a banana tree has a most distinct sound.

THE QI OF CRYSTALS

Crystals have two major energetic functions. Lead glass crystals diffract energy, which is useful for breaking up strong flows of energy and distributing the energy within an area. Mineral crystals contain strong Qi because of the intense heat and pressure under which they were formed. The main purpose of mineral crystals is to introduce additional Qi into areas that are deficient in Qi (a dark, poorly lit room that is seldom used, for instance). While all mineral crystals add Qi, the effect of the Qi varies depending on the mineral; rose quartz introduces Yang Qi effects, while amethyst introduces Yin Qi, for instance.

THE QI OF MIRRORS

Mirrors have a similar effect to lead glass crystal, but their action is limited to reflecting energy. Within a house mirrors can be used to bring pleasant images inside (if your window overlooks a pleasant view or garden a mirror can be positioned so that you can see the reflection of this view from parts of the house where this view would not otherwise be visible.) Placed externally on a house, mirrors can reflect negative or strong flows of energy away. Surrounding a mirror with a Ba Kua sign strengthens its ability to reflect. Flat Ba Kua mirrors simply reflect, convex Ba Kua mirrors diffuse the strength of energy, and concave Ba Kua mirrors neutralise energy by inverting the image.

Mirrored wardrobe doors in bedrooms are powerful movers of energy because they cover such a large area. This can disrupt sleep patterns, especially children's.

RELATIONSHIP QIGONG

Kung Fu Tze had much to say about the various duties and obligations owed to each other by various units of the family, which are also reflected in the overall social structure. Lao Tse also had much to say on this subject in the *Tao Te Ching*, but he was less concerned with duties, obligations and social structure and more concerned with the development of core beliefs such as compassion, honesty and integrity—not as standards which we try to adhere to but as instinctive, spontaneous responses. It could be said that the followers of Kung Fu Tze expressed a yang view of relationships, and Lao Tse expressed the yin approach. As usual, most Chinese people sought to balance the two approaches within their daily lives.

Relationships range from parent and child to husband and wife, worker and boss, teacher and student, guru and acolyte, friend and friend, etc. Qigong techniques relating to the development of the sexual aspects of relationships have been well absorbed in the west, and many books on this subject are available. Other Qigong techniques, such as those applicable to management and government, are less well known and applied.

Relationship Qigong focuses on the fact that your Qi is influenced by those you relate to, and vice versa. Seek relationships that support the Qi of all those involved. This results in a net gain of overall happiness. In a sense, relationships possess their own Qi, and if the Qi of any of the participants is being damaged or adversely affected, the Qi of the relationship will eventually enter a Si Qi or Sha Qi condition. That is, the relationship will either wither or blow apart. The more the relationship contributes to the happiness of those involved in it, the longer it will last and the more value it will provide.

HOW TO APPROACH RELATIONSHIP QIGONG

As with any Qigong, the first step lies in making an assessment of where your relationships are energetically. Then you will be able to establish the direction you want to move in.

Some people may feel that there is not enough 'relationship energy' in their lives. Others may find that their lives are totally dominated by their relationships. Insufficient relationship activity can be due to a lack of social contacts or an inability to 'grow' social contacts into various relationships. This suggests that we need to put more energy into activities that create social contacts or take a closer look at our contacts and identify those may have the potential develop into happy, mutually beneficial relationships.

Too much relationship activity can be attributed to the number of relationships we are involved in or the intensity of individual relationships. You may need to consider terminating those relationships that are not contributing to the happiness of both parties. In the second instance, lower the intensity of those relationships that are causing conflict and emotional turmoil but still have the capacity to contribute to the happiness of both parties.

THE RELATIONSHIP BANK ACCOUNT

Relationships should bring happiness to all parties involved, but it should be recognised that the needs and capacities of participants in relationships change over time. Regard a relationship as a bank account of relationship energy—you 'put in' more when you can and 'draw out' more when you need it. In this way relationships can carry people through the tough times.

CHOOSING RELATIONSHIP PARTNERS

In choosing your home you probably seek the best place that you can afford. If you were offered a house in an area that is run down, has high crime levels and a poor health record, you would think very carefully about the impact it may have on your life. We are not nearly as careful about ensuring that the people we mix with are people who are going to 'enhance' our Relationship Qi. This does not mean seeking out people who can benefit our social or financial position—it simply means seeking out people who expand our ability to achieve our human potential. If we are going to closely associate with people who are constantly negative, angry or depressed, we must also associate with people who have a positive, calm and joyous outlook on life—that way we have a mixture of positive and negative relationships and our relationships collectively are balanced.

SELF-ACTUALISING QIGONG

The process of self-actualisation stems from our need to grow and develop, and to achieve our own potential. When we are on this path we are naturally happy. When we are not, we feel suffocated and confined. If we fail to pursue our human potential, we become depressed, listless and inactive, or we seek activities that coarsen, desensitise and brutalise our inner selves.

Determining the direction that our human potential lies in—let alone actually pursuing that potential—seems such an awesome task that many of us avoid the issue and busy ourselves with basic practicalities of getting on with everyday life. However, one way or another we are always moving closer to, or further away from, our human potential. We have the choice of leaving this to chance, or turning to Qigong techniques that we can apply to assist us on this journey.

Just as human potential varies incredibly from one person to the next, so do the paths that one may take to achieve this potential. Artistic Qigong, Healing Qigong and Recreational Qigong are good starting points, but you may well find others more suited to your individual needs.

ARTISTIC QIGONG

The purpose of Artistic Qigong is not to produce an immortal work of art, but to increase the happiness of the individual through achieving Qi Yun, or 'spiritual resonance', with the universe. Traditionally, Chinese art used the act of creativity to get the artist's energy 'in tune' with that of the universe. The artwork produced under such conditions also had the potential to reveal these 'tunes' to others.

From a Chinese perspective, when we are 'in tune' with the universe we resonate with its internal rhythms and express those rhythms within what we do and create. When the Chinese talk of Tao they are talking about these internal rhythms. Tao is creative by its very nature, so when we are being creative we reflect the basic nature of Tao. This is what makes Artistic Qigong such a powerful technique.

THE TECHNIQUES OF ARTISTIC QIGONG

To get 'in tune' with the universe, traditional Chinese artists did not rely on personal artistic genius, but rather spent hours or even days preparing themselves, physically, mentally and emotionally before creating the artwork. They sought to create the state of Wu Chi within themselves—this being in one sense an emptiness, tranquility and calmness, and in another sense, 'the pregnant void', or source from which everything is born.

Posture, breathing, the materials and techniques used and the environment in which the art was to be created were all considered important in maintaining that resonance with the universe. The artist was more like a 'bridge' between the universe and what the artwork revealed about the universe than a creator of 'art'.

The artist did not seek to express an 'intellectual message', but to generate an artwork that had the capacity to reveal the inner processes of the Tao. In that sense both the artist and any subsequent viewer of the art would be brought closer to being 'in tune' with the universe through a physical, mental, emotional or spiritual response, or a combination of all these.

As in most Taoist techniques, this required great balance on the artist's part. The yang side of art required technique and the application of skill. The yin side of art involved intuition and spontaneity. Like yin and yang, these are opposing but complementary processes. The artist must be careful not to bury spirit with technique, and not to allow spirit to overwhelm technique.

ARTISTS EAST AND WEST

It is interesting to compare the Chinese and western concept of 'the artist'. In the west, the artist is almost expected to suffer poverty, deprivation and frustration before the artwork is finally born from the 'pain' of the creative process. Western artists have rarely been noted for their happiness, whereas Taoist artists were particularly noted for their enjoyment of life. The Taoist poet Li Pai (who is admired almost as much for his untimely end as for his poetry) is one example. Out boating on a lake one night he was so overcome with the beauty of the moon's reflection that he fell out of the boat and drowned while trying to gather the reflection in from the water!

WE ARE ALL ARTISTS

The majority of us probably think our involvement with art is limited to being a 'consumer'. The concept of Artistic Qigong is quite different. The objective of Artistic Qigong is to use the creative act as a means of increasing our spiritual resonance or 'in tuneness' with the universe. Thus while we usually associate art with the creation of a picture or a piece of music, a poem, a piece of calligraphy, a dance—or in fact any action—can be art. The Chinese and Japanese have refined the making of tea to an art. A western parallel to this may be the making of wine. The preparation of a meal can be an art, as can the creation of a garden or the act of arranging flowers in a vase. There are endless opportunities and areas in which to practise Artistic Qigong.

The creation of artwork can be seen as the yang side of Artistic Qigong, and the consumption of art can be seen as the yin side of Artistic Qigong. There is a world of difference between acquiring art and appreciating art. We can buy a CD and play the music, but we cannot appreciate the art it contains until we actually listen to it with the music at the centre of our attention. Likewise, a picture can hang on a wall for months, but it is not until we look at that picture with our full attention that we can be said to be practising Artistic Qigong.

Mindfulness is the end of a process that begins with posture, breathing, and proper preparation of the environment. It leads to Qi Yun. Mindfulness is equally important in the creator of the art and the perceiver of the art.

SHUDAO—THE WAY OF WRITING

While the use of characters—particularly as a way of communicating messages to the gods—has existed for thousands of years, it was not until the third and fourth centuries AD that the art of writing really came into its own. The fact that the Chinese language has pictographic origins adds an extra dimension of meaning to calligraphy. Even the sequence of strokes may influence the nature of the final composition of the character. Thus, a character may convey both a literal meaning and a symbolic meaning. The nature of brushwork adds another level of meaning—it has long been said that a master calligrapher can evoke natural forces such as the manner of wild geese cruising in the sky and beasts running in fright.

Each of these levels of meaning interact, so many messages and thoughts may be carried within one line of writing. This makes any attempt at directly translating traditional Chinese writing virtually impossible.

You will often see Chinese writing across Chinese paintings because writing is seen as an art in itself, capable of conveying as much insight and revelation as a painting. In English writing, each thought and sentence builds on another in a linear sequence. In a very real sense, however, Chinese writing is composed like a picture and one entire thought with all its literal, emotional, symbolic and spiritual meanings is held and released through a whirling stream of brushstrokes. The rational mind cannot contain and hold all of this for release at the same moment, so the artist must use the 'mind within the mind' to unleash the creative energy that lies within. This is why Chinese calligraphy is held in esteem as an artform that can reveal as much to the writer as it does to the reader.

In the west, handwriting experts believe each person's writing is unique. From it they are able to make accurate assessments about the writer's character and psychological state, however bland or meaningless the words. Chinese calligraphy goes one step beyond this, and states that handwriting is but a reflection of the spirit, emotion and thought of the writer at one point in time. Because they are aware that they are revealing their selves for the world to see, Chinese calligraphers take great care to prepare themselves before executing an artwork, to ensure the fullness and purity of the energetic message that they are committing to physical form. Likewise, the reader must be calm and properly prepared if they are to perceive this energetic message in fullness and purity.

CHINESE PAINTING

Chinese painting can often be regarded as a part of the same 'inkplay' as calligraphy. Some styles of painting are even restricted to the same eight basic brushstrokes used for writing Chinese characters.

To practise painting as an Artistic Qigong you do not need to use a Chinese brush and inks or choose Chinese subjects—it is only important that you achieve Qi Yun. First, still the mind, then consider your environment—be tranquil, relaxed and contemplative. Find the state of Wu Chi. The actual creative act must be free-flowing, which requires good posture, lack of muscular and mental tension, and a willingness to 'ride the wind'.

Colours were used in some traditional Chinese paintings, but because the range of colours available was quite limited, colour was not a chief source of expression within the painting. Instead, the painters often focused on landscapes and sought to capture the underlying energetic nature of their surroundings.

MUSIC

Music is the art of organising or arranging sounds into meaningful patterns or forms involving pitch, harmony and rhythm. It is therefore more than 'playing' music on a 'musical instrument'. On first glance it may seem that non-vocal music carries very little meaning, but this depends on whether you think emotional and spiritual meaning exists, as well as intellectual meaning. If 'patterns of sound' carry such meaning, then what exactly is sound? How does it carry meaning and how do we use sound as a Qigong?

What we perceive as sound is actually 'pressure waves' travelling through matter. Our ears detect a transient energy pattern in the matter around us and encode this in the form of electrical impulses for our brain to interpret. When we hear 'language' the brain translates the 'words' into information. Often, however, the information is not carried by words but by the tone, pace and strength of the voice that spoke them. Recordings of the electrical firing patterns that music creates within our brains show that these patterns resemble the firing patterns our brains have when we experience moods such as sadness and joy. This is an awesome thought. A simple pressure wave in the air molecules around us can reveal and create our deepest emotions, our most sensitive moods, and our state of wellbeing.

While our hearing system translates 'sound' to neural impulses, the pressure wave that is the sound travels through every cell in our body. Research shows that these waves can either enhance or detract from the most basic physiological functions of living things, such as cell division. This effect is not restricted to living things either—pressure waves can also support or inhibit inanimate physical processes including chemical and atomic interactions such as those involved in the process of crystallisation.

Many different cultures have recognised the power of music to change the heart and spirit of a person, and singing, chanting and music are often associated with religious practice. In Qigong 'music' is used to achieve Qi Yun or resonance with the universe. Seek out music that makes you feel as if you are in harmony with the universe. Not just music created by instruments, but also the soft 'sighing' of the breeze in trees and grasses and the 'laughing' of mountain streams. We should also think of our own vocal music and let our hearts 'sing' within the words that we speak.

DANCE

FEELINGS ARISE WITHIN US AND MAY BE EXPRESSED IN THE FORM OF WORDS. IF WORDS DO NOT SUFFICE TO EXPRESS OUR FEELINGS, WE SIGH. IF SIGHING FAILS, WE SING. IF SINGING IS NOT ENOUGH, WE EXPRESS THEM BY DANCING WITH OUR HANDS AND FEET.

So says the *Shi Jing* (Classic of Poetry) written some 2700–3200 years ago, even then recognising the close relationship between sound and dance. Throughout history people have generally danced to music. The link between mood, emotion, spirit and dance is very close. We are more likely to want to dance when we are high-spirited and joyful than when we are sad and depressed.

The definition of dance is difficult. We know when we are doing it because of the feeling of energy that is released. To practise dance as an artistic Qigong one must follow the same principles that we have applied in all other Qigongs.

BONSAI AND SUSEKI

Bonsai (the Japanese word for the Chinese art of Pen T'sai) is the art of capturing the large within the small—of creating a tree or a forest only inches high that captures the energy of a huge ancient tree or forest. Why should such an art be a Qigong? To create a bonsai one must 'sense' the energy of the tree and express that energy through the shaping of the tree. The development of this mindfulness and energy sensitivity requires the application of Qigong principles. Like Michelangelo, bonsai artists must seek to discern and release the form that lies within. Unlike Michelangelo, however, who took away the excess stone, bonsai artists must not only prune away but also guide new growth. It is a yin-yang process.

Susukei is the art of selecting and presenting rocks and stones that capture the energy of mighty mountain ranges, rivers, streams and islands, or even living things such as flowers and animals. Again, their collection and display requires one to refine one's awareness of Qi.

The arts of Bonsai and Susukei can be combined to create miniature landscapes. Flower arranging is another way of developing sensitivity and awareness of Qi.

THE ART OF TEA

Tea drinking can be an artistic Qigong. The Japanese ceremony the Cha No Yu is probably the most well-known expression of this artform, but the Cha No Yu was based on Chinese Taoist tea ceremonies. Perhaps the major differences between the Japanese and Chinese tea ceremonies are that the Chinese Tea ceremony is less ritualistic and formal than the Japanese Tea ceremony. Also, a Taoist Chinese tea ceremony must contain laughter for it to be considered successful.

Both tea ceremonies seek to develop a high level of sensory awareness and appreciation, which is essentially the process of Qi Yun. The location of the tea ceremony, the quality of the implements used, the quality and taste of the tea, the sound of the boiling kettle, the aroma of the tea, the fire that heats the kettle, the awareness of all movement and thought that takes place during the tea ceremony—these are the keys to Qi Yun.

HEALING QIGONG

All Qigong heals. Western society tends to make a strong distinction between professional healers and the rest of society. This ignores the fact that much 'healing' is done within the family or community—in particular the cuts, scratches, stomach-aches, bruises, grazes, colds, sniffles, aches, pains, headaches, mental lows and constipation with which the human race is afflicted from time to time. Of course as we have noted before, healing is not just the negative aspect of dealing with injury or sickness; it is also the positive aspect of achieving one's physical, mental, emotional and spiritual potential.

While the healing of more serious conditions must be directed by a professional healer, as a society we are increasingly recognising that healing requires the multi-modal approach of the individual, professional healers, friends and family.

THE HEALING TOUCH

Humans have developed techniques to wreak fearful injury on one another through the use of their hands, but they have also developed techniques that can turn these same hands into healing tools of great efficacy. Every culture and age of history makes some reference to therapeutic touch. These range from purely mechanistic techniques such as Swedish massage to faith-healing, where the healing power is attributed to God or achieving a union with universal forces present in the natural universe.

Traditional Chinese medicine regards all disease and sickness as an imbalance of energy or Qi. An imbalance can be caused by incorrect diet, posture or movement, environmental factors or societal stress. Long-term treatment involves correcting these factors, but if they cannot be removed, or if short-term assistance is required, touch can be used to alleviate the problem.

Touch, in the form of various massage and pressure techniques, may be used to release muscular stress and improve blood circulation. Such techniques can also restore proper Qi flow within an area. Touch also initiates the 'relaxation response', which then contributes to:

- LOWERING BLOOD PRESSURE.
- LOWERING THE VISCOSITY OF THE BLOOD (WHICH IS THICKENED IN THE STRESS RESPONSE).
- REDIRECTING BLOOD SUPPLIES FROM THE MUSCLES TO THE INTERNAL ORGANS SUCH AS THE SMALL INTESTINE TO ASSIST DIGESTION.
- REDIRECTING THE ENERGIES OF THE BODY TO SUPPORT THE IMMUNE FUNCTION AND THE GROWTH AND REPAIR OF THE BODY.

Qigong techniques also use Qi itself to overcome blockages and support deficient Qi flows. In this respect Qi is like water. If you put additional water into a channel it will sometimes wash away an obstruction that was blocking the channel or clear out the channel so that it will flow more easily. This is true whether you are working on yourself or on others. The reason that you can use it on yourself is because you are bringing one part of your body's energetic system into contact with another part.

The use of touch and pressure techniques goes back far into our evolutionary history. The importance of touch cannot be overstated. If all the basic needs of a baby monkey are met but it is deprived of being 'touched', it will die. Human beings appear more resilient, but nevertheless, there is much evidence to show that in situations where touch is eliminated, development is stunted and severe psychological consequences ensue.

HEALING TOUCH TECHNIQUES

The following healing touch techniques are safe and easy to perform. However, if you are pregnant or have had recent surgery, illness or accident, seek medical advice before using acupressure/massage techniques. You should always take care to ensure that rings, jewellery and long nails do not cause injury. Remember that these techniques are used to maintain health and vitality—they may assist in curing certain conditions but you should never dispense with existing treatments. If you wish to know about more healing touch techniques, refer to another of my books, *Dragon Qi Massage*.

Because this is Qi massage, posture, breathing, focused awareness and appropriate environment are important aspects. Don't expect to derive much benefit if you practise these exercises watching TV in a slouched position while constantly being disturbed by family members.

ACUPRESSURE/SELF-MASSAGE FOR THE HANDS

Six organ meridians and one extraordinary meridian are located in the hands. A large number of acupressure points and a complex pattern of reflexology zones are also associated with the hands. Thus you can work on the health not just of the hands but of the entire body by working on this area. The following acupressure techniques are designed to balance and harmonise the flow of Qi within the body without requiring knowledge of the position of key acupressure points or the direction and location of the meridians.

- •- PLACE PALMS TOGETHER. PUSH THE HANDS GENTLY BACK AND FORTH SO THAT THE PALMS RUB GENTLY OVER EACH OTHER. ALLOW THE FINGERS TO INTERLOCK WITH GENTLE PRESSURE. DO THIS FOR 2 MINUTES.

- •- CIRCLE THE PALMS OVER EACH OTHER, MAKING SURE THAT YOU COVER THE WHOLE OF THE PALM, THE FINGERS AND THE WRIST CREASE OF EACH HAND. DO THIS FOR 2 MINUTES.

- •- CONTINUING THE CIRCLING MOVEMENT, ROLL YOUR RIGHT HAND OVER SO THAT THE FRONT OF YOUR LEFT HAND MASSAGES THE WHOLE OF THE BACK OF THE RIGHT HAND. CONTINUE THIS FOR 2 MINUTES THEN REPEAT THE MASSAGE ON THE BACK OF THE LEFT HAND FOR 2 MINUTES.

- •- TAKE YOUR LEFT WRIST AND WRAP YOUR RIGHT THUMB AND FIRST FINGER AROUND IT SO THAT THE THUMB AND FINGERS CIRCLE THE WRIST AT THE WRIST CREASE. THE REMAINING FINGERS OF THE RIGHT HAND LIE ALONGSIDE THE FIRST FINGER, COVERING THE LOWER FOREARM. ROTATE THE LEFT WRIST BACKWARDS AND FORWARDS, APPLYING A FIRM BUT GENTLE PRESSURE WITH THE ENCIRCLING THUMB AND FINGERS FOR A PERIOD OF TWO MINUTES. REPEAT THE PROCEDURE ON THE RIGHT WRIST FOR 2 MINUTES.

- •- USE THE RIGHT THUMB PAD TO MASSAGE THE AREA IN THE CENTRE OF THE INSIDE FOREARM, PUSHING DOWNWARDS FROM THE WRIST CREASE TO ABOUT FOUR FINGERWIDTHS BACK ALONG THE FOREARM. APPLY GENTLE PRESSURE WHEN PUSHING THE THUMB FORWARD AND PULLING THE THUMB BACK IN POSITION FOR THE NEXT STROKE. REPEAT 12 TIMES THEN REPEAT THE PROCEDURE WITH THE LEFT THUMB ON THE RIGHT FOREARM.

- Take your left hand in the tiger's mouth (the area between the inside edge of the thumb and the adjacent edge of the forefinger) of the right hand. The thumb should be on the palm side, pointing in the same general direction as the fingers. The tiger's mouth should enclose the wrist crease. Rub the tiger's mouth backwards and forwards from the wrist crease to the tip of the little finger. Use slight pressure as you move from wrist crease to fingertips. (The thumb pad presses against the palm and inside of the fingers on the left hand. The inner side of the right hand fingers press the back of the hand and the outside of the left hand fingers). Repeat 20 times, then repeat the procedure on the right hand 20 times.

- With the same technique, cover the centre of the palm (the Pericardium meridian and Lao Gong acupoint) and the wrist (an important area of the Lung meridian.)

- In a similar manner, use the tiger's mouth to massage the area between the thumb and first finger of the left hand. Place the thumb pad on the fleshy area adjacent to the back of the thumb, with the side of the first finger adjacent to the lifeline on the palm. Roll the hands to gently massage the fleshy area between the thumb and forefinger for about 1 minute, then repeat this procedure on the right hand.

- Take the base of the thumb of your left hand between the thumb and fingertips of your right hand. As you slowly move your right thumb and fingertips to the top of your left thumb, gently rotate the right hand over the flesh of the left thumb. Under no circumstances should you twist the left thumb joint itself. As the thumb and finger pads reach the lower edges of the thumbnail, stop rotating the right wrist backwards and forwards and apply firm pressure against the lower corners of the thumbnail with the pads of the thumb and forefinger. Now release the left thumb by 'flicking' the thumb and forefinger off the left thumb.

- Repeat this procedure on the left thumb 3 times, then perform the same process on each of the fingers of the left hand 3 times. Repeat the entire procedure on the thumbs and fingers of the right hand. Any pressure you apply must be gentle. On no account should there be any strain on the joints of the digit.

ACUPRESSURE/SELF MASSAGE FOR THE HEAD AND FACE

Because the head and face are situated in the most yang part of the body, the massage techniques used in this area are usually those that have a relaxing and calming effect. Stress, congestion of sinus and navel cavities, yang headaches, irritability and muzzy thinking can be reduced by massage in this area. The ears also relate holistically to many other areas of the body.

- PLACE BOTH HANDS AGAINST YOUR FACE WITH THE FINGERTIPS POINTING UPWARDS, ROUGHLY IN LINE WITH THE NOSE. PUSH THE HANDS UPWARDS, ALLOWING THE INSIDE OF THE FINGERS AND THE PALMS TO PLACE A GENTLE PRESSURE AGAINST THE FACE. CIRCLE THE HANDS OUTWARDS AND DRAW THEM DOWNWARDS ALONG THE OUTSIDE OF THE FACE UNTIL THE FINGERTIPS REACH THE CHIN. CONTINUE THE CIRCLING MOVEMENT UPWARDS, OVER THE LIPS AND UP THE SIDES OF THE NOSE, RETRACING THE PREVIOUS PATH. COMPLETE SIX FULL CIRCLES, MOVING SLOWLY AND APPLYING GENTLE PRESSURE.

- EXTEND THE CIRCLE BY PUSHING THE FINGERS UPWARDS OVER THE TOP OF THE HEAD, MAINTAINING GENTLE PRESSURE ON THE SCALP AND DRAWING THE HEELS OF THE HANDS DOWNWARDS, BEHIND THE EARS, ACROSS THE THROAT AND UNDER THE JAW TO MEET. BEFORE THE FINGERTIPS LOSE CONTACT WITH THE NECK, PUSH THEM UPWARDS OVER THE CHIN AND LIPS AND ALONG THE SIDES OF THE NOSE TO CONTINUE THE CIRCLE. REPEAT 6 TIMES.

- PLACE THE THUMB PADS BEHIND THE APEX OF THE RIM OF EACH EAR. GENTLY PRESS THE OUTSIDE RIM OF EACH EAR BETWEEN THE THUMBS AND FOREFINGERS. MAINTAINING GENTLE PRESSURE, DRAW THE THUMB AND FINGER DOWN THE RIM OF THE EAR AND ACROSS THE EARLOBE, PULLING THE EARLOBE DOWNWARDS AND OUTWARDS WITH COMFORTABLE PRESSURE. REPEAT THIS MOVEMENT 6 TIMES.

- RUB THE HEELS OF THE HANDS TOGETHER VIGOROUSLY UNTIL THEY ARE QUITE WARM. CLOSE YOUR EYES AND PLACE THE WARM HEELS OF YOUR HAND GENTLY AGAINST THEM SO THAT THE HEAT AND QI WARMS THE EYE. REPEAT 3 TIMES.

ACUPRESSURE/SELF-MASSAGE FOR THE ABDOMEN

The abdomen is another area that is holistically related to the rest of the body. Acupressure work in this area affects our digestive and eliminative systems, improves the blood supply to all of the internal organs located in this area (the Tan Tien), which is one of the most important energy storage areas of the body. The massage outlined below is one of the most important acumassage techniques used in China. Practise this massage once a week for three weeks and you will notice that your digestive and eliminative functions are running better and that you have more energy, alertness and wellbeing.

- Begin in a standing or sitting position, with a straight spine and relaxed shoulders. Breathe through the nose and visualise each breath penetrating deep into the abdomen. Place your left hand on the lower abdomen so that the palm rests just inside the right pelvic bone. Place the right hand on top of the left hand. Keep the shoulders relaxed.

- Press down gently as you move the hands upwards to a point just under the rib cage. Maintaining gentle pressure, pull the hands across the top of the abdomen just under the rib cage. Push the hands downwards along the left side of the abdomen to a point just inside the pelvic bone, then pull them across to the right hip, back to the starting point. Finish by bringing the hands to a point just under the navel. Repeat this circling of the abdominal area at least 36 times.

To perform this movement as Qigong, breathe in as you move your hands up and across to your left side and breathe out as you bring your hands down and across to your right side. While performing the exercise, visualise a beam of energy extending into the abdomen from your left palm as it moves and stirs the contents of your abdomen. As this is a Qi massage movement, being mentally focused is more important than whether or not you are applying pressure. Be sure to maintain an upright position and always move in the direction described above, which follows the natural movement of the digestive process along the ascending, transverse and descending colon. Avoid this exercise if you have just eaten a large meal or if you have diagnosed abdominal problems.

MIND POWER QIGONG

The mind and body are like the two sides of a thin sheet of paper. It is virtually impossible to do anything to one side of the paper without affecting the other side. We now recognise how important physical exercise is to all parts of the body, including the muscles, joints, ligaments, tendons and tissue. Most of us are also familiar with the vast number of exercise forms that can be used to develop and maintain the body. With respect to exercise of the mind, we have developed the ability to store more facts faster and have improved our analytical and computational skills, but we are largely unfamiliar with the need to 'exercise' the emotions and spirit. We are also unaware of the basic techniques that can be used exercise and develop theses areas.

'Healing mind techniques' include positive affirmation, visualisation, biofeedback and meditation. While each of these techniques has a useful role, meditation best serves the purpose of a Healing Qigong. In meditation the mind focuses on sensory input such as a sound, a sight, a smell, the kinaesthetic awareness of the body, or some other external object.

QI MEDITATION

Qi meditation uses the power of the mind to influence the circulation and transformation of Ren Qi within the body. By focusing the mind on key energy centres and flow patterns within the body, the flow of Qi can be balanced and harmonised. In Qi meditation we focus on the familiar areas of environment, posture, breathing and mental focus.

THE MEDITATION ENVIRONMENT
Your surroundings should be quiet and pleasant, free of distracting sounds, draughts and extremes of temperature. The air should be fresh and have a pleasant aroma. The light should not be too bright. Clothing should be loose and comfortable. Meditate at a time when you are not likely to be disturbed and are under no time pressure.

POSTURE
Qi meditation may be practised sitting on a chair or in standing position. Lying down is not recommended, as it is better to have the spine in a vertical position. If sitting, the feet should be placed flat on the floor with the upper leg horizontal and the lower leg vertical. Kneeling, lotus-type postures, and cross-legged positions are not recommended.

BREATHING
The flow of your breath should be relaxed, natural and diaphragmatic.

MENTAL FOCUS
Using the mind, follow the focus on each specific acupoint and meridian and visualise yourself 'leading' Qi.

OPENING UP THE MICROCOSMIC ORBIT

The microcosmic orbit is the name given to the energy pathway that is formed by the Du Mai and Ren Mai meridians. This is the prime energy circuit of the body. The acupoints situated on this meridian are listed on page 152.

- - • - ACHIEVE THE CORRECT MENTAL FOCUS BY VISUALISING A GLOWING GOLDEN SPHERE ABOUT THE SIZE OF A GOLF BALL SITUATED AT THE SHENQUE ACUPOINT. MAINTAIN THIS VISUALISATION FOR APPROXIMATELY 5 MINUTES.

- - • - PICTURE THE SPHERE MOVING SLOWLY DOWN TO THE NEXT MEDITATION POINT LISTED IN THE TABLE ON PAGE 152 AND AGAIN HOLD THE VISUALISATION FOR A PERIOD OF 5 MINUTES.

- - • - CONTINUE ON IN THIS MANNER UNTIL YOU HAVE PASSED THROUGH ALL THE LISTED POINTS. THIS WILL RETURN YOU TO THE SHENQUE POINT, WHERE YOU SHOULD THEN VISUALISE THE SPHERE DIFFUSING BACK INTO THE ABDOMINAL AREA.

It is important to follow the points in the order given. If you have to interrupt the meditation, move your imaginary sphere through the other points without pausing until you reach the Shenque point, where you should pause to imagine the sphere diffusing back into the abdomen before terminating the meditation.

If you encounter unpleasant or disturbing sensations during a Qi meditation, re-centre your energy at the Tan Tien. If the symptoms are particularly disturbing or do not diminish with practice, seek advice from a Qigong expert.

After you have practised the full microcosmic orbit daily for a month or so you may like to progress to the macrocosmic orbit.

MEDITATION POINTS OF THE MICROCOSMIC ORBIT

Shenque	Immediately behind the navel
Qi Hai	Three fingerwidths below the navel
Guan Yuan	Two fingerwidths above the pubic bone
Qugu	At the upper border of the pubic bone
Hui Yin	In the centre of the perineum (between the anus and the genitals)
Yao Shu	2.5cm up from the tip of the coccyx (tail bone), in the hiatus of the sacrum
Ming Men	Between the first and second lumbar vertebrae
Zi Zhong	Between the eleventh and twelfth thoracic vertebrae
Feng Fu	At the base of the skull
Bai Hui	The very centrepoint of the top of the crown
Yin Tang	The midpoint between the eyebrows
Su Liao	At the tip of the nose
Tian Tu	In the notch of the bones at the base of the throat (technically, the centre of the suprasternal fossa)
Shan Zhong	In men in the centre of the chest, level with the nipples. In women about 3cm above the base of the sternum, technically on a level with the fourth intercostal space.
Zhong Wan	Four fingerwidths above the navel
Shenque	Immediately behind the navel

MEDITATION POINTS OF THE MACROCOSMIC ORBIT

Shenque	Immediately behind the navel
Hui Yin	In the centre of the perineum (between the anus and the genitals)
Wei Zhong	In the centre of the back of the knees
Yong Quan	On the soles of the feet at the junction of the anterior/middle sole
Yin Bai	On the big toe, just below the bottom of the toenail root
Da Du	Extends along the inside edge of the foot to the joint of the lower bone of the toe
He Dig	Top of the knee
Hui Yin	In the centre of the perineum (between the anus and the genitals)
Ming Men	Between the first and second lumbar vertebra
Da Zhi	Between the spinous process of the seventh cervical vertebra and the first thoracic vertebra
Qu Qi	On the outside end of the elbow crease when the arm is flexed
Lao Gong	In the centre of the palm
Wai Guan	On the back of the wrist, three fingerwidths from the crease
Da Zhi	Between the spinous process of the seventh cervical vertebra and the first thoracic vertebra
Bai Hui	The very centrepoint of the top of the crown
Shan Zhong	In men in the centre of the chest, level with the nipples. In women about 3cm above the base of the sternum, technically on a level with the fourth intercostal space.
Shenque	Immediately behind the navel

ALSO BY THIS AUTHOR

Feng Shui for Personal Harmony 2000
Living Chi Simon & Schuster 1999
Tai Chi for Better Breathing Simon & Schuster 2001
Tai Chi for Stress Control Simon & Schuster 1993
Tai Chi—the Way to a Healthy Life New Holland 2000

Grandmaster Gary Khor is the Founder and President of the Australian Academy of Tai Chi and Qigong, and the Feng Shui Academy of China.
website: www.livingchi.com.au
e-mail: aatc@optushome.com.au

NOTE

Throughout this book the terms BCE (before common era) and CE (common era) correspond with BC and AD.

ACKNOWLEDGEMENTS

I wish to thank David Walker for his tireless work in the research and development of ideas for this book, and its final proofreading while I was in China. My gratitude also goes to Master Zen Feng for his patience and ever willing assistance. My sincere regards to Professor Lim of the Kwangsi province of China for his kind advice and consultations over the years. And finally, my thanks and appreciation to those at New Holland especially Jennifer Lane for her meticulous effort in editing the text and Nannette Backhouse for her great graphic work.

Gary Khor

INDEX

First published in North America in 2004 by Weatherhill, Inc.,
by special arrangement with New Holland Publishers.

Published in Australia in 2004 by
New Holland Publishers (Australia) Pty Ltd
Sydney • Auckland • London • Cape Town
14 Aquatic Drive Frenchs Forest NSW 2086 Australia
218 Lake Road Northcote Auckland New Zealand
86–88 Edgware Road London W2 2EA United Kingdom
80 McKenzie Street Cape Town 8001 South Africa

Printed in Singapore

Publishing Manager: Robynne Millward
Project Editor: Jennifer Lane
Designer: Nanette Backhouse
Production Manager: Janelle Treloar
Reproduction: Colourscan, Singapore
Printer: Tien Wah Press (Pte) Ltd, Singapore

ISBN 0-8348-0545-6

10 9 8 7 6 5 4 3 2 1

Picture credits

NANETTE BACKHOUSE (GRAPHICS): pages 23, 24, 25, 27,
30, 32, 34-5, 41, 52, 53, 54-5, 99, 100-1, 120, 122, 129, 142,
144-5, 148, 149.
ESTHER BEATON: pages 12, 13, 19, 49, 50, 91 (bottom),
92 (top), 94 (bottom), 102, 118-119.
IAN FAULKNER (ILLUSTRATION): pages 37, 38, 72-3,
74 (top and bottom), 75 (top and bottom), 76.
GETTY IMAGES: front cover, pages 14, 16-17, 77, 90, 91 (top),
93 (top and bottom), 95, 112, 113, 114, 134-147.
GARY KHOR: pages 22, 28-9, 36(original article), 64, 67, 68, 69,
78(original), 82, 86, 92 bottom, 97(original), 125(original),
128(original), 141(original).
DANNY KILDARE: pages 20, 21, 26 (all three), 58, 62, 78, 84,
88, 94 (top), 97, 104-5, 106-107, 121,125, 126, 127, 128, 139,
141, back cover (centre).
NEW HOLLAND IMAGE LIBRARY (NHIL): pages 39, 43, 44,
81, 130, 131, 132, back cover (top and bottom).
SCIENCE PHOTO LIBRARY: pages 6, 7, 10, 11, 46.